The Aesthetics of Senescence

SUNY series, Studies in the Long Nineteenth Century
———————
Pamela K. Gilbert, editor

The Aesthetics of Senescence

AGING, POPULATION, AND THE
NINETEENTH-CENTURY BRITISH NOVEL

Andrea Charise

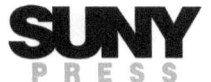

Cover image: Thomas Rowlandson. "Medical dispatch or Doctor Doubledose killing two birds with one stone." Published by Thomas Tegg, London, 1810. © The Trustees of the British Museum. All rights reserved.

Published by State University of New York Press, Albany

Published in cooperation with the University of Regina Press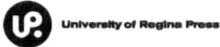

© 2020 State University of New York

All rights reserved

Printed in the United States of America

No part of this book may be used or reproduced in any manner whatsoever without written permission. No part of this book may be stored in a retrieval system or transmitted in any form or by any means including electronic, electrostatic, magnetic tape, mechanical, photocopying, recording, or otherwise without the prior permission in writing of the publisher.

For information, contact State University of New York Press, Albany, NY
www.sunypress.edu

Library of Congress Cataloging-in-Publication Data

Names: Charise, Andrea, author.
Title: The aesthetics of senescence : aging, population, and the nineteenth-century British novel / Andrea Charise.
Description: Albany : State University of New York Press, 2020. | Series: SUNY series, studies in the long nineteenth century | Includes bibliographical references and index.
Identifiers: LCCN 2019005904 | ISBN 9781438477459 (hardcover : alk. paper) | ISBN 9781438477466 (pbk. : alk. paper) | ISBN 9781438477473 (ebook)
Subjects: LCSH: English fiction—19th century—History and criticism. | Aging in literature. | Old age in literature.
Classification: LCC PR868.A394 C43 2019 | DDC 823/.809354—dc23
LC record available at https://lccn.loc.gov/2019005904

10 9 8 7 6 5 4 3 2 1

Nature's vast frame, the web of human things,
Birth and the grave . . . are not as they were.

—Percy Bysshe Shelley, "Alastor; or,
The Spirit of Solitude," 1816

Contents

List of Illustrations		ix
Preface		xi
Acknowledgments		xv
Introduction: The Aesthetics of Senescence		xix
Abbreviations		xlv
Chapter 1	William Godwin and the Artifice of Immortality	1
Chapter 2	"In the condition of an aged person": Mary Shelley and Frail Romanticism	33
Chapter 3	George Eliot's Aging Bodies	63
Chapter 4	"The Century's corpse": Reading Senility at the *Fin de Siècle*	101
Chapter 5	Writing Twenty-First-Century Aging Populations	141
Notes		151
Works Cited		167
Index		185

List of Illustrations

Figure I.1   Anonymous. "The various ages and degrees of human life explained by these twelve different stages."   xxxix

Figure 1.1   William Blake. "Aged Ignorance." From *For the Sexes: The Gates of Paradise*.   9

Figure 2.1   William Heath. "Burking poor old Mrs Constitution Aged 141."   43

Figure 2.2   Thomas Rowlandson. "Medical dispatch or Doctor Doubledose killing two birds with one stone."   43

Figure 3.1   Pieter Breughel the Elder. "Misanthrop" [The Misanthrope].   82

Figure 3.2   William Blake. "London." From *Songs of Innocence and of Experience: Shewing the Two Contrary States of the Human Soul* [Songs of Experience].   86

Figure 3.3   William Blake. "The Ecchoing Green" [recto, Plate 1, and verso, Plate 2]. From *Songs of Innocence and of Experience: Shewing the Two Contrary States of the Human Soul* [Songs of Innocence].   88–89

Preface

Early in the process of writing this book, I proposed to my department that I develop a seminar for our advanced undergraduates. Called "Reading Older Age," its goal was to introduce students to representations of age and aging in a variety of literary genres, to better understand how such portrayals contribute to our perceptions of fleshly temporality. An obvious place to begin the curriculum, I thought, was with Matthew Arnold's 1867 poem "Growing Old":

> What is it to grow old?
> Is it to lose the glory of the form,
> The lustre of the eye?
> Is it for beauty to forego her wreath?
> —Yes, but not this alone.

The teacherly tone of Arnold's opening question, I hoped, would prompt my students (all in their early twenties) to articulate exactly what growing old meant to them. I was right. Their answers—"frailty," "65," "white hair," "Alzheimer's," and (my favorite) "cataracts and prune juice"—clearly expressed what age theorist Margaret Gullette describes as the "ideology of decline" (*DTD* 7), that is, the naturalized assumption that old age is inextricably bound to illness, incapacity, lack, and diminishment. This did not inspire much confidence in what I could achieve in a semester to counteract or even complicate such ideas. But the seminar continued and, in the final class, I asked my students once again to reflect on Arnold's question. This time, after twelve weeks of reading a spectrum of literary engagements with aging, older age, and late style (texts ranging from Shakespeare's *King Lear* to David Markson's *The Last Novel*), those same readers for whom old age had been a largely insensible idea generated reflections that were considerably more complex and inventive than the first day's. I was struck by the outcome of this unintentionally Wordsworthian exercise: by reading for age in and through literature, together we had begun to see into the life of things.

My own interest in the literary study of older age is prompted by nearly two decades of health research, primarily in geriatrics. In fact, I began working in geriatrics at about the same age as my undergraduates. Several years later, I decided to pursue graduate studies in English Literature, examining representations of old age in nineteenth-century British writing. Well-meaning inquirers from both medicine and literature found this puzzling: their response, when I told them, was usually a "What?" accompanied by a compensatory gesture (a tilted head, or a cupped ear), almost invariably followed by a baffled "Why?" I suppose it is no big mystery why the study of older age is perceived as somewhat unseemly. In the twenty-first century, there is much about older age that can feel off-putting or even repulsive. Gerontologist Harry Moody sardonically terms older people "the ill-derly" (135), referencing both literature and health policy's stubbornly ageist conflation of aging with senescence and death—filled with dreadful visions of dementia and physical decline. This antipathy is a major barrier for the field of Age (or "Aging") Studies, and for its researchers. It effectively brands the investigator of aging as peculiar, or even perverse; it is weirder still, apparently, when a younger scholar chooses to undertake such a study, like the eccentric aged child of a Dickens or Hardy novel. Reflecting on my own experience, the clearest indication of such aversion was expressed not so much in the mystified "Why?" but in the failure or reluctance to give ear to the words "old age" in the first place.

Since then, things have changed—at least in part. Age Studies is experiencing an ascendance in the form of professional networks of scholars in Europe and North America, major academic publications, and annual guaranteed convention panels at the Modern Languages Association. Literary and cultural critics such as Kathleen Woodward, Karen Chase, Devoney Looser, Stephen Katz, Teresa Mangum, Helen Small, Kay Heath, Thomas Cole, and Margaret Gullette have been instrumental in establishing the formal, thematic, and activist aims of the field. I am myself thoroughly indebted to these colleagues and other scholars.

My objective, in this book, is to extend and amplify this vital conversation. The novels I have chosen to examine here are drawn from a wide array of modes: gothic and speculative, pastoral, realistic, and naturalistic. I do not promise an exhaustive survey of a theme or complete genealogy of a phenomenon, nor should my selections suggest that the novels I discuss mark to the exclusion of all others decisive flashpoints in the history of thinking about older age during this period. Instead, I have chosen to focus on texts that exemplify what I see as especially interesting or provocative moments in the nineteenth-century imagination of older age, precisely because they re-present the profound multivocality of aging and older age at the moment of their textual production. The work continues.

In his 1925 thesis on German tragedy (later published as *Origin of the German Trauerspiel*, 1928), philosopher Walter Benjamin famously compared the relationship between ideas and their material expression to an astronomical constellation: a configuration that both groups together individual stars and is revealed by their cluster. Benjamin's image is a valuable one in the context of my project, and of Age Studies in general. In many ways, the idea of "what it is to grow old" can only be conceived of as a motley assemblage of definitions, bodily symptoms, language, and representations, none of which, on their own, can be held up as fully exemplary. This is as true for health professionals as it is for literary critics and laypeople. Aging is not this or that alone, as Arnold recognized. In place of merely cataloguing instances of literary representation (an irksome critical mode I call "spot the old person"), my interdisciplinary approach aims to identify this constellatory essence of older age in the nineteenth-century British literary imagination and, importantly, in our own time as well. Just as the handle of one celestial cluster points to the belt of another, so the manifestation of an idea in one age points to its expression in another. As readers, we must not only be guided by these signals; we must also consider how they interact, and how they might be reconceived—a bright star abandoned for one that is not yet seen.

Acknowledgments

This book was shaped by my doctoral studies at the University of Toronto, where I was encouraged to conduct interdisciplinary research as a PhD candidate in English and the Collaborative Program in Health Care, Technology, and Place. While I was there, Alan Bewell, Cannon Schmitt, and Elizabeth D. Harvey were exemplars of generous, challenging, and respectful mentorship. I am profoundly grateful for their confidence in the initial phases of this work, and to have had the chance to learn alongside them.

With the support of a fellowship from the Social Sciences and Humanities Research Council of Canada, my work continued as a postdoctoral researcher at the Obermann Center for Advanced Studies at the University of Iowa. Hearty thanks to Teresa Mangum, Director of the Obermann Center, for some of my fondest memories of writing, researching, and developing ideas in such an intellectually generative, supportive, and sustaining environment. I am honored to have received the John Charles Polanyi Prize for Literature as a result of the new avenues opened up by my postdoctoral experience.

Sometimes it is possible to point to a decisive moment in one's life where one path diverges from another. For me, it was the opportunity to work in the Division of Geriatric Medicine at Parkwood Hospital, London, Ontario, in my early twenties. I owe a significant debt of gratitude to the geriatricians who first encouraged my research in aging and nurtured my interests in arts-based health research—in and among all of the clinical care, education, and advocacy they do on a daily basis on behalf of older people: Drs. Laura Diachun, Jennie Wells, Monidipa Dasgupta, and Michael Borrie, as well as Judy McCallum and Wendy Parisian. You have my lasting admiration and thanks.

More recently I have had the support of outstanding colleagues in the Interdisciplinary Center for Health & Society at the University of Toronto

Scarborough (UTSC), including Holly Wardlow, Jessica Fields, Michelle Silver, Suzanne Sicchia, and Cassandra Hartblay. Thanks also to Paul Stevens, Linda Hutcheon, Katie Larson, Michael Lambek, Karen Weisman, Ian Balfour, Terry Robinson, Danny Wright, David Francis Taylor, Michael Trussler, and Michelle Flax for their sage advice and heartening insights.

I have been lucky enough to get a sneak peek at the next generation of teachers, scholars, and activists in the fields of Age Studies (and Health Humanities more generally) in the form of my marvelous undergraduate students, past and present, at UTSC; I am so excited to see how you will transform our collective experience of aging in the years to come. My experience working with graduate students in University of Toronto's Graduate Department of English has been a precious source of joyful intellectual exchange; I have especially appreciated the energetic provocations of Dimitri Pascaluta, Olivia Pellegrino, Katherine Shwetz, Stefan Krecsy, and Nicole Dufoe, who taught me how to read what I thought were familiar things, anew.

Colleagues in the North American and European Networks of Aging Studies have been encouraging from the early days, especially Margaret Morganroth Gullette, Stephen Katz, Kathleen Woodward, Erin Gentry Lamb, Sally Chivers, Pia Kontos, Cynthia Port, Ulla Kriebernegg, Tom Cole, Valerie Lipscomb, Leni Marshall, Aynsley Moorhouse, Julia Gray, Danny George, Andy Achenbaum, and Peter Whitehouse. I have found genuine community among a range of Health Humanities associations, including the Health Humanities Consortium, International Health Humanities Network, and the Modern Languages Association's forum on Medical Humanities and Health Studies. Special nods to Paul Crawford, Tess Jones, Rebecca Garden, and Nehal El-Hadi for the flourishing interdisciplinary nuclei they have established and continue to foster.

Deep appreciation goes to SUNY Press for their interest in this book, especially Amanda Lanne-Camilli, Acquisitions Editor, and Pamela Gilbert, "Studies in the Long Nineteenth Century" Series Editor. My thanks to Jenn Bennett-Genthner, Production Editor, and Fran Keneston, Director of Publicity & Marketing, for shepherding the manuscript into book form; copy editor James Harbeck for his careful review of the finer details; and Ellen L. Hawman for synthesizing a thoughtful and comprehensive index. My appreciation extends to the University of Regina Press—Karen May Clark, Duncan Campbell, and Jonathan A. Allan especially—for producing an exquisite Canadian English-language paperback edition of this book. Anonymous readers helped improve the manuscript via their thoughtful and encouraging commentary; special credit is due for this crucial yet invisible task. I promise to pay it forward.

I had the chance to articulate an initial draft of my prefatory remarks in "The Future is Certain: Manifesting Age, Culture, Humanities," *Age, Culture, Humanities: An Interdisciplinary Journal* 1 (2014), pp. 11–16. Much earlier segments of the introduction and chapter 2 appeared in the article "Romanticism Against Youth," published in *Essays in Romanticism*, vol. 20 (2013), pp. 83–100. A version of chapter 1 first appeared in *English Literary History (ELH)* 79.4 (2012), pp. 905–933, as "'The tyranny of age': Godwin's *St. Leon* and the Nineteenth-Century Longevity Narrative." Chapter 3 grew out of a short conference paper, "G.H. Lewes and the Impossible Classification of Organic Life," published in *Victorian Studies* 57.3 (2015), pp. 377–386. Bits of chapter 5 first appeared in "'Let the reader think of the burden': Old Age and the Crisis of Capacity," *Occasion: Interdisciplinary Studies in the Humanities* 4 (2012), pp. 1–16. Thanks to these journals for their support of my research throughout the process.

My friends and family: here you are, once again, last in the order of things. Pascale McCullough Manning and Stewart J. Cole have long brought light and love in ways that warm me daily. To the oldest and best, I say: *champagne?* I am blessed that my loving and relentlessly optimistic kin—Michael, Victoria, David, Alicia, Phillip, and each of my grandparents—have been extended by fortune to include the Tysdals and the Falls. And to Daniel who, for the past thirteen years, has expanded and recombined my life with trust, courage, imagination, and happiness: I admire your work. This book is for you.

Introduction

The Aesthetics of Senescence

Recent years have witnessed the publication of alarming yet familiar headlines: apocalyptic visions of an imminent "grey" or "silver tsunami" of aging retirees (*The Economist, The Globe and Mail*); a "lost generation" of unemployed younger workers (*The Atlantic, Huffington Post*); and even a "war against youth" (*Esquire Magazine*). The common thread of these reports is their assumption of an inherent incompatibility between age-based cohorts—a belief reflected not only in the popular media, but in public policy and scholarly research as well. How has chronological age come to possess such far-reaching ideological, ethical, and aesthetic repercussions? How did age-based identities coalesce into such fraught realities? And how did Matthew Arnold's question "What is it to grow old?" describe an evidently pressing problem for a diverse range of nineteenth-century British writers? In this book I argue that authors of this period used the imaginative resources of literature to engage with an unprecedented—and, as in our present day, hotly politicized—climate of crisis associated with growing old.

Two related watershed events occurred at the close of the eighteenth century, with the publication of books by leading thinkers of the day. One was philosopher William Godwin's hugely popular *Enquiry Concerning Political Justice and its Influence on Modern Morals and Happiness* (1793). The other, which first appeared anonymously in 1798, was titled *An Essay on the Principle of Population as It Affects the Future Improvement of Society, with Remarks on the Speculations of Mr. Godwin, M. Condorcet, and other Writers*. (The English cleric and scholar Thomas Robert Malthus did not openly acknowledge authorship of his incendiary book until the larger second edition appeared in 1803.)[1] The two writers' ideas were widely influential, yet Godwin's radical idealism was quickly eclipsed by Malthus's clear-eyed critique, which took particular umbrage with Godwin's declaration of the possibility of human life lived without end. Because their competing sets of ideas, known as the 1798 Godwin-Malthus debate, involved a profound shift in emphasis—from the individual life to the "massified" framework of population—their writings transformed not only the nature of the human subject but also, I argue, the very meaning of fleshly temporality.[2]

Godwin's *Political Justice* (reprinted with significant edits in late 1795 and again in 1798) consistently asserted that old age was nothing less than the embodied symbol of political tyranny; and that radically prolonged life was the material sign of a truly free humanity. But after Malthus's devastating critique of such idealism, Godwin's hopes evidently broke down. Within a year, Godwin's next novel examined exactly what the lived consequences of immortality might actually mean not only for an individual but for society as well. Following the success of his first novel, *Things as They Are; or, The Adventures of Caleb Williams* (1794), in Godwin's *St. Leon: A Tale of the Sixteenth Century* (1799), the titular hero—granted everlasting youth by a magic elixir—lives beyond the ordinary span of life only to discover that this unnatural state separates him from the rest of humankind, even those closest to him. As I argue in chapter 1, Godwin's second novel is important because it constitutes the first example of what I call the nineteenth-century "longevity narrative"—presenting an extreme case of age as a conditional state, rather than a stage, of life, one conceived specifically in relationship to the lived reality of an aging population.[3]

With its theme of the necessity of individual decline, in order to fuel the collective perpetuity of life, *St. Leon*'s startling reversal of a key facet of *Political Justice*'s philosophical radicalism illustrates a broader cultural reassessment of the paradoxical necessity of old age to human progress. It is also symptomatic of a broader shift away from Enlightenment perceptions of human lifespan as limited, limiting, and incarceral (as in Rousseau's claim in his *Confessions* book VIII, that he "was born in a dying state" [95]), and toward a new cognizance of the role played by bodily decline. As a speculative case study of an unbounded life that turns out to be, in fact, disastrous, *St. Leon* signals an acute transitional moment in the early nineteenth-century politics of generation. Godwin explores the social compatibility of youth and age across a variety of disciplines: his historical novel blends elements not just of literature, but also of philosophy, medicine, economics, and fantasy, to produce a complex epistemological investigation of age, aging, and the ideological lineaments of senescence itself.

I discuss both these writers in more depth later, but for now, suffice it to say that the 1798 Godwin-Malthus debate inaugurated a new biopolitics of lifespan. A book like this could approach the subject by pointing to well-known catalysts of social change during this period: the French Revolution, industrialization, the rise of empire, and so on. My study, by contrast, asserts that a new conceptualization of human aging, and the thoroughly refigured bodies it gave rise to, constituted a major cultural upheaval in itself. I employ the language of biopolitics as a useful shorthand for describing how older age was increasingly portrayed as both a *medicalized* and *politicized* bodily state. *Medicalized* in the sense of attracting new forms of authoritative knowledge concerning human health (as per the hypothesis articulated by social theorists like Ivan Illich in *Medical Nemesis* (1976), for example); and *politicized* in the sense of such knowledge emerging as an issue of both public and private health concern (typically associated with the work of Michel Foucault, or later elaborations such as Barbara Ehrenreich's *The American Health Empire: Power, Profits, and Politics* (1971) and *Natural Causes: An Epidemic of Wellness, the Certainty of Dying, and Killing Ourselves to Live Longer* (2018)). This shift, I propose, marks a transition away from the primarily religious thinking of earlier historical periods, toward one that made strategic use of decidedly literary ways of knowing about aging. At this time of profound cultural upheaval, the imaginative capacity of writing became an interdisciplinary crucible for testing what it meant—or could mean—to grow old. Motivated by concerns that are alive and well in our own time, this book is about the reorientation of the meaning of aging following the introduction of population as a character in the early-nineteenth-century British cultural landscape. To return to Arnold's question, perhaps my aim is less to define "what it is to grow old" in nineteenth-century Britain than to illustrate how that century—its literature, science, politics, and culture—was radically transformed by growing old.

While modern literary criticism has, over the past three decades, thoroughly embraced the study of class, race, gender, and sexuality in the formation of individual, social, and literary subjects, less attention has been paid to the role of age as an integral element of identity. The field of Age Studies, in its broadest sense, exists to describe the critical study of the interlinking concepts of age (the chronological number of years a person has lived), aging (the ongoing temporality of the body, including mental and physiological changes often associated with post-midlife), and older age (a vague, context-dependent designation generally starting at sixty-five years of age). As defined by Margaret Gullette, Age Studies takes as "its founding proposition, the priority of culture in constructing age . . . [f]rom the confetti of the phenomena to the confetti-factories of ideology" (*DTD* 106). Aging's compulsory combination of ideology and biology makes Age Studies an intensely interdisciplinary field involving anthropological, psychosocial, historical, materialistic, and humanistic imperatives, "because it emphasizes the language we use, the genres our stories get shaped into, our visual and verbal discourses" (116).

Even studies of old age that are primarily historical—such as Susannah Ottaway's *The Decline of Life* (2004), Pat Thane's *Old Age in English History* (2000), or Simone de Beauvoir's *The Coming of Age* (1972)—routinely cite the relevance of art and literature to shifts in the meaning and experience of growing old. Recent Age Studies work has focused almost exclusively on the Victorian period, emphasizing our interpretation of cultural and historical artifacts. Yet few scholars have investigated the intersection of medical, scientific, philosophical, economic, and demographic discourses around older age as represented in nineteenth-century British writing. This book therefore adopts age, and older age especially, as an *analytical category* of textual study, charting the traffic between literary and extra-literary engagements with human aging, to ask 1) how does the nineteenth-century British literary imagination employ age as a means of identifying certain age-defined populations or cohorts, and 2) in what ways do such attempts reflect, dispute, or even seek to undermine the emergence of demographic thinking during this period? This new, double-stranded question forms the basis of my exploration of the evolving attitudes toward an emergent—and unprecedentedly public—cultural politics of aging and older age in nineteenth-century Britain.

Nineteenth-century demographic data provides further context for this study, as do more modern back-projection techniques that "retropolate" (as opposed to "extrapolate") more granular assessments of societal age structure at that time. From 1801 to 1871, national census data reported an overall increase in England's population from 8.71 million to 21.37 million; in the early nineteenth century especially, population growth was most apparent in rapidly industrializing areas.[4] Between 1780 and 1829 life expectancy at birth ranged from 48 (male) to 55 (female) for the property-owning classes, increasing to 50 (male) and 62 (female) between 1830 and 1879. In addition to significant variations in life expectancy at birth based on class, gender, and location, it is also important to remember that such measures are only partial reflections of demographic reality due to factors like high infant and child mortality rates (which reduced overall life expectancy calculations) (Antonovsky 33). Over a similar period, the percentage of the population aged 60 or older was approximately 5 to 7 percent throughout the century, slightly lower than the 6 to 10 percent cited for the late seventeenth and early eighteenth centuries (an apparent decline primarily due to high birth rates that boosted the population percentage-share of the very young).[5] Then as now, class difference cannot be overstated: in 1838, statistician William Farr identified that the mean life expectancy of the general population was almost twelve years less than that of the peerage (40.4 versus 52 years).[6]

This fundamentally level plateau of life expectancy and overall proportion of older persons changed abruptly in the 1890s, with both measures steeply ascending over the course of the twentieth century. Between the 1890s and 1980s, Peter Laslett writes, the "long term, enduring . . . irreversible" phenomenon he terms *the secular shift in aging* "was so fundamental that it can indeed be conveyed only in geological metaphors . . . transferring the sense of fundamental, physical structure conveyed by the notion of landscape to the architectonics of society" (67). To the extent that the British case reflects broader global trends today, the shift Laslett describes is indeed reaching a new, "loftier" (67) plateau both with respect to life expectancy and proportion of older persons in the developed world. In the United Kingdom 16 percent of the population is sixty-five or older (2011), in Canada 16.9 percent (2016), and in the United States 14.9 percent (2016).[7] Particularly in comparison to the early years of the nineteenth century, recent census data confirms a brave new age of human aging itself. It remains to be seen whether such gains in life expectancy are in fact irreversible in light of twenty-first-century socioeconomic inequalities, environmental threats, chronic illness, and other emergent population-based risk factors.

In *The Shape of Irish History* (2001), A.T.Q. Stewart writes, "The days, weeks, months and years mark out our lives, and we measure time by the customary life-span. A century seems a very long time to us precisely because it is just beyond the normal" (16). Following Godwin's epic experiment, nineteenth-century British literature contributed important strategies for representing what old age was—or might be—in the context of longer life spans not only for individuals but for populations as well. One of the questions I explore is how prominent British writers shaped, witnessed, and represented "the invention of the elderly subject" (as Karen Chase puts it in *The Victorians and Old Age*, 276). Of course, this requires some reading against the grain, since literature of that era typically took youth as its default perspective and subject—from its young protagonists, to marriage plots, to the novel as a form itself. In *The Way of the World: The Bildungsroman in European Culture*, Franco Moretti distinguishes between the hero of the classical epic—a mature man like Achilles, Hector, or Ulysses—and that of the novel (for example, Goethe's *Wilhelm Meister*), which effectively "codifies the new paradigm, and sees *youth* as the most meaningful part of life" (3, emphasis in original). Yet such a perspective has rarely accounted for a considerably more varied understanding of aging throughout nineteenth-century writing, the novel especially. For these reasons, this book considers how the theme of senescence can also help us to analyze the "aging" nineteenth century in new ways. The Victorian response to its precedent Romanticism is one such trope; another might be the insistent rhetoric of "life-course" so often used to characterize the culture and literature of this period. Consider the critical lexicon used to describe this century's literary production: we speak of "proto-Romanticism," and of "first- and second-generation" Romanticism; and then of "early," "mid-" and "late" Victorianism—ending, of course, with the terminal throes of the *fin de siècle*. No other period has generated as detailed an inventory of chronologized stages. Then as now, that century has aged anxiously, and literary scholarship continues to project vivid visions of aging onto it and its textual productions.

My aim in this work is twofold. First, I demonstrate how introducing the concept of "population" as a character into the cultural landscape in the early years of the century helped reconceive older age as a biopolitical state of life; and second, I investigate how nineteenth-century literature, in particular, became an important experimental space for shaping an emergent aesthetics of aging, longevity, life-course, and even life-extension in response to new disciplinary understandings of aging bodies. Regarding the first objective: each chapter explores how senescence became a potent nexus of theory, imagination, and embodiment, provoking a distinctly modern suite of concerns about its implications for both individual and social bodies. Famously, Malthus's invention of demography in 1798 shifted emphasis from individual lives to the framework of population. What are less well considered, however, are the consequences that form the through-line of my study: how this radical reconfiguration of the body politic had profound consequences for longstanding views of human temporality. Before Malthus, aging was conceptualized as a linear progression through ordained "stages"— as recounted, for instance, in Jaques's "Seven Ages of Man" monologue in Shakespeare's *As You Like It*:

> All the world's a stage,
> And all the men and women merely players;
> They have their exits and their entrances;
> And one man in his time plays many parts,
> His acts being seven ages . . . (2.7.138–142)

After Malthus, aging began to acquire an unfamiliar biopolitical overlay. The new consciousness of population recast aging as a *state* of life, fluid and unstable, and inseparable from the broader health and future of society. Contemporary critics including Emily Steinlight, Maureen McLane, and Frances Ferguson have shown that in the same period—which saw the birth of the human sciences such as moral philosophy, political economy, and anthropology—thinkers were profoundly concerned not only with the lives experienced by individuals, but with populations as well. It was the construction of the elderly as an identifiable population that made older citizens newly subject to social discourse, especially as burden, difficulty, or disruption: a pattern of thought readily available in our own day precisely because of its development over the long nineteenth century. By bringing this established research to bear on my investigation of age-based visions of generational identity, my book builds on these discussions to consider the nineteenth-century construction of youth, older age, and intergenerational conflict as matters of not just familial but social and demographic trepidation.

Although generational conflict has long existed as a trope in Western literature (e.g. *Oedipus Rex, King Lear, Mrs. Warren's Profession*), a diverse range of nineteenth-century texts indicate the intimate linkage of the emergent science of demography with shifting perceptions of human age as the flashpoint of social crisis. My second aim in this book is to build on these discussions to investigate how multiple disciplinary paradigms used literary strategies to examine, and appraise, newly medicalized ideas of what it was to grow old. In stark contrast to the Old Testament injunction "Be fruitfull and multiply" (Gen 1.28, King James Bible), a distinctly Malthusian strain of thought identified the thriving reproductive capacities of youth as the catastrophic basis of overpopulation. As chapter 2 describes, the immense backlash generated by such age-based anxieties effected what we might today call a culture war, pitting those hostile to the "juvenile warmth" of post-Revolution Europe (to use politician Edmund Burke's phrasing in the *Reflections*, 213) against those who viewed youth and its aesthetics—championed by literary figures that included, for a time at least, William Godwin, William

Wordsworth, and Percy Bysshe Shelley—as antithetical to the rank inequities of an *ancien régime*. Textual modes of experimentation, and especially the imaginative capacity of literature, afforded a crucial interdisciplinary apparatus through which human aging—its meaning, representational strategies, and symbolic and lived repercussions—could be investigated, tested, illustrated, or even remedied. Such a study further allows us to see that ideologies also live in and through time; in other words, they age. What produces stability and coherence for one generation will not do the same for another, a truth forcefully displayed in the contrast of George Eliot and George Gissing's respective portraits of age and aging in chapters 3 and 4. As the second half of my book lays bare, clearly the images that fed midcentury dreams of older age left hungry those in the *fin de siècle*.

Interpreting the history of aging populations is a comparatively recent investigation. Yet equally germane is the matter of disciplinary methods: how was the aging body apprehended at the dawn of that century? In our own time, fields of research, academic departments, and funding agencies are rigorously segregated. More often than not, so-called "interdisciplinary" initiatives merely serve to reinforce the trend toward hyper-specialization: they engage only fields that already share assumptions, narratives, and vocabularies (literature and history, for example, or medicine and nursing). The recent emergence of initiatives like "narrative medicine" or "Health" (also "Medical") Humanities marks a significant attempt to articulate, and occasionally bridge, such disciplinary and epistemological fissures. (Of course, the very act of doing so—as required when proposing interdisciplinary courses, securing research funds, building a tenure file, or writing a book—indicates the conceptual distance that still persists to separate these fields of interest.) But in the nineteenth century, these realities were not nearly so pronounced. Then as now, the concept of aging was a particularly good example of this multidirectional epistemological traffic. *The Aesthetics of Senescence: Aging, Population, and the Nineteenth-Century British Novel* is therefore also about the nature of interdisciplinary exchange between literary and non-literary ways of knowing at that time, habits of thinking that reveal themselves as newly germane to our understanding of similar issues in the twenty-first century.

The Malthusian Intervention

To set the stage for my argument, I will briefly examine the intellectual context of England and Europe before Malthus published his *Essay* in

1798. Before then, the sheer proliferation of human bodies had long been knit to positive indices of social and national prosperity. Throughout the early modern period, for example, the prevailing mercantile system directly linked a nation's political and economic power to the size of its working population. Growth was actively encouraged by laws that penalized celibates and made marriage a prerequisite for holding public office. Yet despite such official endorsements of reproduction, the reality was that the destitute class was growing ever larger. In 1601, the English Poor Laws were introduced at the parish level to provide relief (money, food, clothing, and so on) to paupers and to those too ill or debilitated to work. Within a century, the British population had increased to such a degree that these policies had to be revised and Europe was witnessing an explosion of population literature that would soon challenge the pronatalist ideology of a former era.[8] Clearly, population growth was not interpreted as a universal boon.

One significant controversy, which in some ways presaged the Godwin-Malthus debate of 1798, was the question of whether or not human fecundity had diminished since antiquity. In his 1752 essay "Of the Populousness of Ancient Nations," David Hume contends that in the present, "every wise, just, and mild government, by rendering the conditions of its subjects easy and secure, will always abound most in people, as well as in commodities and riches" (*Essays* 226). In contrast, Hume believed, the dependence of the ancients on slaves, and the draconian restrictions placed on this large class of people, significantly hampered early populations. Robert Wallace's *Dissertation on the Numbers of Mankind in Ancient and Modern Times* (1753) shared the broad ideological contours of Hume's position, but arrived at the opposite conclusion—that the ancient world was in fact more populous than the present. This debate, moot as it was, can be interpreted as a remnant of the seventeenth century's obsession with the decay of nature and the apparent old age of the world. This "melancholy of mutability" (Williamson 121) was a popular motif in the literature, religion, and philosophy of that era, and inspired some of Romanticism's key themes.

The ideas of Hume and Wallace laid the groundwork for more practical studies of population: not just how many people might have lived in the past, but how they might be measured in the present—and forecast in the future. Then, against the mercantilist paternalism of Hume and Wallace, Adam Smith's *An Inquiry into the Nature and Causes of the Wealth of Nations* (1776) rejected the premise that government should engineer economic wellbeing. Smith's *Wealth of Nations* held that population numbers are simply another expression of free market forces, guided by the invisible yet insistent hand of supply and demand: "The demand for men, like that for any other commodity, necessarily regulates the production of men; quickens it when it goes on too slowly, and stops it when it advances too fast" (81). While Smith was appalled by the practice of infanticide (which, he noted in *Wealth of Nations* and elsewhere, was common in China), at home the abstracted hand of demand and supply was nevertheless free to exert its suffocating influence to identical effect.

In fact, Smith cites China as a case study of perfectly balanced, stationary rate of population growth—thereby perpetuating historians' longstanding view of the Orient as an orderly, populous empire. For example, the translator's dedication of French Jesuit historian Jean-Baptiste Du Halde's encyclopedic and widely translated *The General History of China* (1738, 1741)[9] conspicuously praises the country's orderly population control:

> No Laws or Institutions appear in the general so well contrived as the *Chinese* to make both King and People happy. . . . Nations as numerous as the Sands of the Sea are restrained within the Bounds of the most perfect Submission. . . . Hence likewise *China* has but seldom experienced Revolutions, which have so often overturned other States; and were it not for the superstitious Sects that have been suffer'd to propagate themselves, had probably never felt any.

Yet this ostensible situation of "most perfect submission" made some European observers suspect that China's population restraint might be less the embodiment of good government, and more the result of tyrannical and despotic micromanagement. "Might not our missionaries have been deceived by an appearance of order?" wondered Montesquieu in *The Spirit of Laws* (1748) (154). By the late eighteenth century, China's population was estimated to be 300 million (Europe's, by contrast, was some 200 million, and England's a mere 8 million); even there, however, poverty was widespread. Despite his qualms, Montesquieu could not help concluding that Chinese women must be "the most prolific in the whole world" to enable that country to rapidly recover from the regular devastations of famine (155).

As this brief overview reveals, the proliferative nature of populations occupied the Orientalist dreams of European theorists long before Malthus's notorious *Essay*. It was in this intellectual context that *An Essay on the Principle of Population as It Affects the Future Improvement of Society, with Remarks on the Speculations of Mr. Godwin, M. Condorcet, and other*

Writers first appeared anonymously in 1798. The *Essay*'s lucid and original hypothesis still resonates more than two centuries later: the geometric growth of human populations (1, 2, 4, 8, 16, 32, 64, 128 . . .) is limited by merely arithmetical increases in subsistence (1, 2, 3, 4, 5, 6, 7, 8 . . .). Left unchecked, the former will always outstrip the latter. By positing a perpetual struggle between population growth and available resources, the *Essay* conceives nature less as a bountiful and all-giving life force than as a constraint to which humanity is inescapably subject, thereby innovating the concept of "overpopulation."

Malthus articulated two types of checks to population growth: *preventive* ones that lower the birth rate (i.e., late marriage or abstinence) and *positive* ones that raise the death rate (i.e., disease, war, famine). Following breakfast conversations with William Godwin, Malthus also added *moral restraint* (sexual abstinence) to the 1803 edition as a third, if speculative, means of alleviating population pressure. As we shall see in the next chapter, the *Essay* asserts a harsh, temporally dynamic vision of population wholly distinct from the rational, benevolent one of Godwin's *Political Justice*—essentially articulating the bifurcated terms on which conceptualizations of aging would be scaffolded in the decades and centuries that followed.

Rather than limiting its significance to a defense of a hypercapitalist status quo, it is important to note how Malthus's *Essay* targets the fearsome reproductive capacity of youth. In her book *The Body Economic: Life, Death, and Sensation in Political Economy and the Victorian Novel* (2005), Catherine Gallagher astutely observes that in the *Essay*, "Malthus's argument ruptures the healthy body/healthy society homology," and that in terms of population control, "the healthy body comes to be a sign of its opposite" (*BE* 39). Malthus further disrupts the longstanding affiliation of health and youth by introducing a new hermeneutics of lifespan, one that does not equate youth, reproductivity, and the new with unreserved or unqualified benefit. In fact, old age—rather than an antagonist to progress or a pathology requiring eradication—instead connotes a surprising indicator of individual and national fitness. In an unusually figurative passage describing the American colonies (a newly forged nation, through Eurocentric eyes, following the 1775–83 War of Independence), Malthus imagines the body politic in terms of the inexorability of both population growth and aging:

> A person who contemplated the happy state of the lower classes of people in America twenty years ago would naturally wish to retain them for ever in that state, and might think, perhaps,

> that by preventing the introduction of manufactures and luxury he might effect his purpose; but he might as reasonably expect to prevent a wife or mistress from growing old by never exposing her to the sun or air. The situation of new colonies, well governed, is a bloom of youth that no efforts can arrest. There are, indeed, many modes of treatment in the political, as well as animal, body, that contribute to accelerate or retard the approaches of age, but there can be no chance of success, in any mode that could be devised, for keeping either of them in perpetual youth. (114–115)

By acknowledging one's "natural" tendency to "wish" for an eternally favorable misfit between population and resources, Malthus anticipates a reader sympathetic both to Enlightenment ideals of perpetuity and to mercantilist assumptions of ceaseless increase. The sad truth, Malthus is obliged to inform us, is very different—as illustrated by his rhetorical migration from the tentative "would" and the conditional "might" to the harsh realism of the indubitable "is." Prior to Malthus's intervention, commentators such as Smith, Godwin, and Benjamin Franklin had noted with admiration the flourishing of the North American colonies. Food, jobs, and land were plentiful and it was widely remarked that human numbers had doubled in twenty-five years. Malthus checks this happy attitude by glimpsing in North America's "well-governed" growth cause for grave concern.[10]

This passage is remarkable for the many ways it overturns the meaning of population growth as an axiomatic social good. Key to his rhetorical strategy is the language that emerged from the late eighteenth century's taxonomic imagination. As Amy M. King observes in *Bloom: The Botanical Vernacular in the English Novel* (1998), Carl Linnaeus's investigation of the sexual function of plants gave rise to a "botanical vernacular" that made it possible to mention female maturation in both literary and non-literary writing of this period. Writers from Jane Austen to Henry James were able to reference a woman's "bloom" as a shorthand for her sexuality, in a way that King characterizes as both "explicit (as it is in Linnaean systematics), and safely implicit" (5). The metaphor of bloom, she points out, is "a mediating figure par excellence: a figure than can traverse the range from innocent to provocative, and that can bridge the accepted social appearances of courtship with the specifically physical manifestations of maturation and enticement" (5).

Malthus, however, employs the metaphorics of bloom against its newly sexualized tenor to warn against a foreboding youthful fertility that "no efforts can arrest." In a strikingly paternalistic metaphor of commodification, Malthus compares the lower classes to "a wife or mistress" whom the (naturally male) reader would "wish" to keep in a state of unmarred allurement. Malthus undercuts those fond hopes precisely because they defy the sequelae of this crucial organic metaphor (perhaps an insight planted by the melancholic Jaques of *As You Like It*: "from hour to hour we ripe and ripe, / And then from hour to hour we rot and rot" [2.7.26–27]). Hereby hangs the *Essay*'s sober tale: rather than a sign of good government, sexual bloom directly competes with the agricultural bloom vital to food production and subsistence. In opposition to pronatalist enthusiasts, for Malthus the value of bloom is stubbornly attached to its literal associations with farming and agriculture. Although cosmetic delays are possible, population growth—like bodily aging—retains its devastating inevitability. Bodily bloom is thus the grim augur of a withering nation.

The passage quoted above, in fact, marks the crux of what Gallagher calls Malthus's "double vision" of the body-nation analogy. As she observes, "the social body is growing 'old' precisely insofar as the actual demographic proportions of society are increasingly weighted toward youth . . . The social body is an 'old woman' insofar as it is populated by young women" (*BE* 39). Malthus's conclusion—that there is "no chance of success" for keeping either the political or the physical body "in perpetual youth"—reveals the semantic extent of this double vision of youth and age (Malthus 115). He further observes that, "by encouraging the industry of the towns more than the industry of the country, Europe may be said, perhaps, to have brought on a premature old age" (115). The use of "premature" is telling here. The *Essay* describes an inverse relation between the health of a population and the reproductive capacity of the bodies it contains. But this also signals that Gallagher's assessment of the social body as at once "growing old" and being "an old woman" requires some refinement. Recall Malthus's acknowledgment that some interventions "may contribute to accelerate or retard the approaches of age" (115): Europe's *premature* old age announces that the effective age of the nation is less a function of chronological time than of its rate of population growth. Malthus says as much when he explains, "the happiness of a country does not depend, absolutely, upon its poverty or its riches, upon its youth or its age, upon its being thinly or fully inhabited; but upon the *rapidity* with which it is increasing" (55, emphasis added). For

Malthus, it is the temporal and bodily instability implied by the process of aging—and not the state of old age *per se*—that presents the real threat to happiness. The procreative "success" of youth merely ushers in the disastrous outcome of its realization.

From this we may therefore assume that "aging," "growing old," and "old age" are not equivalent terms in the *Essay*, nor ought they be conflated in more general discourse—as Age Studies theorists have argued. "Two words—*age* and *aging*—cover and blur too many separable ideas," writes Margaret Gullette (*DTD* 212). Margaret Cruikshank, in *Learning to Be Old: Gender, Culture and Aging*, likewise observes that it is not "the changes in our bodies that define 'old'; it is the meanings given to those changes" (5). Whereas "old states" such as Europe, France, or England are less prone to vacillations from stability to misery, national aging is concurrent with the rapid and dynamic change that accompanies the treacherous march of progress. Paradoxical as it may sound, in the Malthusian view premature national aging—that is, the too-rapid increase in youthful bodies—is the worst of both worlds: it incorporates both the vulnerability of old age, and the proliferative instability of youth. The ideal state, we might suppose, would be one that possesses the stability of the old without passing through—to borrow Mary Poovey's apt and inadvertently Malthusian phrase—the "nightmare of . . . maturity" (153). (In chapter 2 I investigate how this peculiar circumstance might play out.)

Malthus also articulates a concept new to the nineteenth century, which we might now term *ephebiphobia*—a coinage that describes the fear or dislike of youth, while also carving out a surprising admiration accorded to older age, as a check to reproduction. Malthus further challenges the assumption that the female body is the *sine qua non* of population growth: while not exactly perpetual, the male capacity to reproduce lasts at least for most of the lifespan. This striking formulation points to the need to refine Gallagher's assessment of the "predictably" feminized social body she ascribes to Malthus's *Essay* (*BE* 39), which seems to place Malthus back within a mercantilist paradigm. By contrast, defying the ancient stigma associated with the menopausal body, Malthus takes a positive view of older women—precisely because they "are beyond the potential to multiply" (Niles, "Malthusian," 295). The diminished female fecundity associated with menopause informs Malthus's observation that female misery—namely illness and violence—acts as a check to population.

This assessment is consistent with his controversial comparison of the fertile woman and the childless spinster (added to the *Essay*'s second edition of 1803). Speaking of a hypothetical "matron who has reared a family of ten or twelve children," Malthus warned against "the character of the monopolist" in this ostensibly "great benefactor to the state." The "old maid," in his view, "on the contrary has exalted others by depressing herself.... She has really and truly contributed more to the happiness of the rest of the society arising from the pleasures of marriage, than if she had entered in this union herself." By remaining childless, the spinster has a better "claim to the gratitude of society" than a mother (148–149). No great imagination is required to imagine the widespread outrage this passage provoked; Malthus expunged it from the third (1806) edition.[11] But despite the controversy they generated, Malthus's ideas caught on in some circles: echoes of them are manifest in, for instance, the writings of Jane Marcet (*Conversations on Political Economy*, 1816), Harriet Martineau (*Illustrations of Political Economy*, 1832–1834), and novelist Elizabeth Gaskell.[12] The old maid—be it through body or behavior—acts as a calming salve to the population crisis begotten by youth.

To modify Gallagher's claim that population pressure in a society depends only on the number of women of childbearing age, Malthus insists that young men as well—the elect of savage and civilized nations alike—compose a formidable reproductive class whose mobility, especially in times of war and political unrest, makes them the primary agents of an ever-threatening apocalypse. Male fecundity is dangerously coupled to other enticements and tendencies feted in bawdy war songs. For example, the Chevalier de Boufflers's "Love and War" (translated by poet and essayist Leigh Hunt in 1824) views the human losses of combat in lockstep with zestier duties when it rallies, "What possible debtor can pay his debts better, / Than De-population with Re-population?" (Hunt 329–330). Turning to the working class, a laborer who is unprepared to support the reproductive consequences of his vice (that is, having children) "may in some respects be considered as an enemy to all his fellow-labourers" (Malthus 44); as with the fecund woman, his fecundity serves as a symbol of the antisocial logic at the basis of species generation. By introducing masculinity as a dangerous "aging" factor for the nation, Malthus effaces the traditional gendered view of population growth as solely a female responsibility.

For this reason, Malthus considers the three groups of women, children, and the aged as posing the least risk of increasing the population; and he identifies increases in the numbers of these groups as the best way to gauge the health of a nation. This contrasted with the former general tendency to focus on young men—"gentlemen-warriors" in their prime of life—as the best indicator of social vigor:

> In estimating the happiness of a savage nation, we must not fix our eyes only on the warrior in the prime of life: he is one of a hundred: he is the gentleman, the man of fortune, the chances have been in his favour; and many efforts have failed ere this fortunate being was produced. . . . The true points of comparison between two nations seem to be the ranks in which each appear nearest to answer to each other. And in this view, I should compare the warriors in the prime of life with the gentlemen, and the women, children, and aged, with the lower classes of the community in civilized states. (Malthus 28)

In Malthus's view, the lives of women, children, and the elderly are usually risked—and often sacrificed—to preserve the young male demographic. Old and young, male and female, rich and poor, civilized and savage, the old world and the new: youth trumps them all, an internal enemy with the potential to destroy the fragile balance between population and resources.

The *Essay* thus adopts a Blakean trope when it divides old and young into contrary states, effectively pitting youth against age, the former a natural enemy of the other. To be old is to be innocent of enabling the menacing annihilation associated with reproductivity, a state to some extent native to the female body given that the inevitability of menopause diminishes fecundity. By defining states of age based on reproductive capacity, Malthus presents a view of society as one of disastrously incompatible warring classes—its social bonds perpetually threatened by youthful bloom: a remarkable because biological reframing of longstanding ideological conceptualizations of age, aging, and older age in Britain and European culture more broadly at this time.

In some ways, Malthus's skepticism also registers the political conservatism of Edmund Burke, whose 1790 publication *Reflections on the Revolution in France* celebrates the stability of "the ancient world" in contrast to the destructive ethos of innovation.[13] Using a suite of gerontophilic motifs, Burke defensively contrasts the revolutionary French with the staid English: "I know that we are supposed a dull, sluggish race, rendered passive by finding our situation tolerable" (203). Yet these qualities, Burke maintains, constitute the very means of ensuring national longevity. His disgust for those who reject the legacy of the past is linked with an overt reverence for the aged: Burke himself was sixty when he wrote the *Reflections*, in "the stiff and peremptory dignity of age" (365), ostensibly addressing his observations to "a very young gentleman at Paris" (151). In this text and others (perhaps most notably five years later, in Burke's spirited vindication of his right to a state pension in *Letter to a Noble Lord*), the intellectual and moral stability of age serves as a rhetorical defense of England's past against a dangerous mania for change. In his view, "juvenile politicians" sympathetic to the French cause err gravely by abandoning the value of "experience and observation" (364):

> Such schemes are not like propositions coming from a man of fifty years' wear and tear amongst mankind . . . These gentlemen deal in regeneration; but at any price I should hardly yield my rigid fibres to be regenerated by them, nor begin, in my grand climacteric, to squall in their new accents or to stammer, in my second cradle, the elemental sounds of their barbarous metaphysics. (364–365)

Burke employs an alchemical trope to defend the "grand" and "rigid fibres" of the past against the "barbarous metaphysics" of revolution, and passionately rejects the political regimen that would make an ideological infant of the man in life's "second cradle." Little wonder that he concludes the passage with a quotation adapted from Cicero's *De Senectute* (*On Old Age*): "*Si isti mihi largiantur ut repuerascam, et in eorum cunis vagiam, valde recusem!*" In the original quotation, Cato the Elder lectures his young colleagues on the benefits and values of later life. Cicero's original text affirms the speaker's contentedness: "If some god should give me leave to return to infancy from my old age, to weep once more in my cradle, I should vehemently protest" (Cicero 95). Burke's adaptation, by contrast, is motivated by a strongly ephebiphobic resistance to embracing the politics of youth in the "second childhood" of old age: "But if those guys [the pejorative pronoun *isti*] should give me leave to return to infancy from my old age, to weep once more in *their* cradle, I should vehemently protest" (emphasis added).[14]

With his *Reflections*, Burke effectively lays the moral and political groundwork for Malthus's physiological ephebiphobia eight years later. In other words, the *Essay* reinvents Burke's dislike for "regeneration" in terms of sexual reproduction; the political risks of innovation and revolution Burke voiced in the *Reflections* become the *Essay*'s fears of youth and population. However, Malthus is no mere biological Burkean. As well as departing from the *Reflections*' overt mercantilism and "Augustan values" (Collings, *Monstrous* 185), the *Essay* also discards Burke's dogged insistence on preservation, sameness, and tradition. For all the *Essay*'s anxieties about youth, Malthus is resigned to the juggernaut of change driven by the catastrophic inevitability of human reproduction. Here lies the essential distinction between Burke's and Malthus's conservatisms: the latter focuses on a *biological* principle of continuity rather than a *genealogical* one. Biology effaces the singularity of ancestry by introducing the vast numbers of population: sexual generation, not ancestry, is the true basis of national history. By expanding the scope of Burke's palpable fear of revolutionary crowds, Malthus recasts this ideological clash of generations as an outright war—while also reserving an unexpected place for older age as a tenuous bulwark against the dangers of reproduction.

The Aesthetics of Senescence

Far from an isolated idiosyncrasy, Malthus articulates distinct anxieties regarding the emergence of age as an ideologically freighted demographic identity. Malthus's immediate impact on language, policy, and cultural discourse cannot be overestimated: in direct response to the 1798 *Essay*'s recommendations, Prime Minister William Pitt the Younger withdrew his support for a parliamentary bill that he had formerly endorsed, which had proposed to enhance monies given to the poor in proportion to family size (Bonar 208). Some of "Parson" or "Pop" Malthus's most vocal detractors included prominent literary figures like Samuel Taylor Coleridge, Robert Southey, and William Hazlitt, who were appalled by the *Essay*'s apparent ruthlessness toward the poor. (Writing in 1836, Coleridge explodes: "Is it not lamentable—is it not even marvellous—that the monstrous practical sophism of Malthus should now have gained complete possession of the leading men of the kingdom! Such an essential lie in morals—such a practical lie in fact as it is too!" [Coleridge, *Table* 88].) Most immediately, these new biopolitics of aging inserted a wrinkle into the prevailing iconography of the deeply Christian architecture of the age-as-stage model. As historian of aging Thomas R. Cole has shown, since the mid-sixteenth century, the dramaturgical language of "stages" has served to describe to the journey of the human body through time. In contrast to the immense divine machinations that gave purpose to the brutishly short medieval existence, the age-as-stage model was visually rendered as a rising and falling staircase known as the *Lebenstreppe* (German; English translation, "steps of life"). Widespread throughout Europe and North America until the early twentieth century, the *Lebenstreppe* presented the bourgeois individual with a conceptual playbill that placed him (or her, or both) at the center stage of his own life-course: an existence now replete with prescribed roles, plot, and temporal projection into the future (see figure I.1). This motif, complete with its predictable plotting of the life-course as a purposeful quest through life's chaos, "provided a visual means for each person to step outside his own life experience and view it as a whole" (Cole 25). The upward ascent of childhood and youth, the peak of man's "perfect age," followed by the downward slope of later years, meant that the journey of modern aging implied by the stages model was as much a spatial as temporal organization of one's life.

In contrast to this age-as-stage model, new concepts of population necessarily influenced, and demanded, aesthetic representations sensitive to new conceptualizations of aging: a model or, indeed, *models* more reflective of affective states and social conditions that were themselves subject to change as both affects and conditions alter. That literary writing, the novel especially, would be responsive to such ideations is consistent with what is known about the nineteenth century's interest in the body as a subject for the literary imagination. Scholars including William A. Cohen, Nicholas

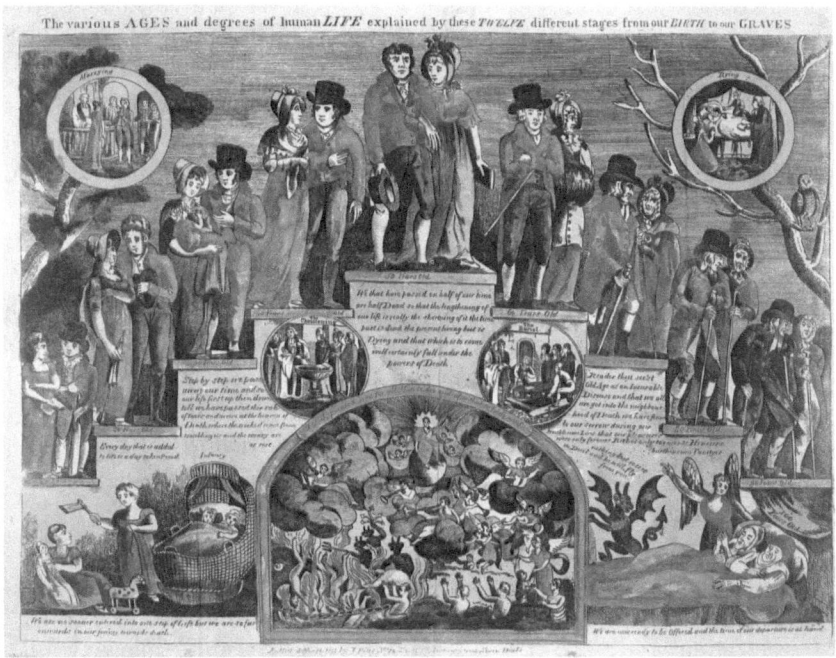

Figure I.1. Anonymous. "The various ages and degrees of human life explained by these twelve different stages." Published by John Pitts, London, 1811. © The Trustees of the British Museum. All rights reserved.

Dames, Gillian Beer, Pamela Gilbert, Athena Vrettos, and Sally Shuttleworth have shown how novelistic representations of corporeal experience are now increasingly understood to inform key modes of representation typical to the novel such as interiority, character, realism, and psychological depth. Nor were bodily sensations purely a matter for literary writing: scientific texts were also informed by an awareness of the physical realm. This intricate interconnection of disciplinary knowledges produced "a loosely affiliated coterie of scientists, journalists, and intellectuals who brought the experimental study of human physiology to bear upon the facts of novel-reading" (Dames, *Physiology* 2). My book extends this significant body of knowledge by focusing on the more and less implicit conversations between medicalized and literary understandings of aging at this time, particularly the ways in which this interdisciplinary traffic complicated conventional notions of human temporality typical to the archetypal linearity of the *Bildungs*-plot. Above all, each chapter is interested in the convergence of aesthetics, disciplinary knowledges, and nineteenth-century British culture as conceptual grounds for the twenty-first century's profound aversion toward and fascination with the facts—and as importantly, the imaginative fictions—of human aging and older age.

Because I am taking a long view of materials produced across Romantic and Victorian periods—two periods of literary history that are often kept apart, somewhat artificially—let me be clear about some key threads and patterns that I am especially interested in tracking throughout this book:

- ***The nineteenth-century British novel as an ideal form for historicizing changing senses of human temporality.*** By reading the novel (the mode of literature that arguably attempts most to do justice to the span of lives—the *Bildungsroman* especially) in conjunction with scientific analyses and philosophical speculation on the rhythms and dynamics of life, I examine how novelistic fiction is uniquely prepared to grapple with the complex heteroglossia of human aging. Numerous characters I will discuss here are indeed "old," but not necessarily, or straightforwardly, in terms of chronological age. Thus I acknowledge and assert the variety of definitions necessary to capture the range of representations discussed in the following chapters, as the assignment of "old" is deployed to describe certain features, behaviors, and actions ranging from clichés and stereotypes to more nuanced and idiosyncratic applications. By situating a literary epistemology in the midst of, or in relation to, other "extra"-literary discourses like medicine, economics, or philosophy, it becomes possible to read these divergences and alignments in strategies for thinking about aging as part of the conceptual and aesthetic structure by which representations of experience are shaped by human temporality.

- *Nineteenth-century British writing on aging as the stage for dynamic tensions between secular and religious notions of lifespan.* As described above, the dominant ages-and-stages model of life was intimately informed by a Christian—and, often, Protestant—paradigm. While lifespan is not exactly a doctrinal issue, there nevertheless exists a range of figures, parables, and stories that convey what old age is or looks like, how it relates to earlier phases of life and, perhaps most importantly, a sense of the afterlife that survives more or less vestigially into the nineteenth century. The introduction of population as a framework for conceiving of human life was itself inseparable from religious discourse (Malthus was, after all, a cleric of the Church of England), but it also signaled a departure from the lingua franca of Christianity. Recent understandings of the relationship between secular and religious thought during this time recognize that secular scientific and/or medicalized thought was not nearly as divorced from Biblical or religious paradigms as today's readers might suppose. The portraits of aging and older age that I discuss here become an opportunity to track in what ways the novel, novelists, and less apparently literary writers might still rely on putatively displaced models of religious thought—even as secularized visions of aging began to gain traction.

- *The translation of physical laws into aesthetic principles that scaffold the imagination of aging and older age.* Gravity, entropy, erosion, and volumetrics are examples of physical properties and laws that shape the way nineteenth-century aging appears in the literary and extra-literary texts of this time. Perhaps above all, the matter of capacity—how many years a body can (or should) hold, how many people (old, young, or otherwise) a society can accommodate—becomes an urgent and highly influential matter of concern in the wake of population-based thinking, particularly at the *fin de siècle*. Such concerns underpin more twenty-first-century articulations of what Kathleen Woodward has recently called "statistical panic," which describes intensely affect-driven responses to the apparent indisputability of proclamations concerning disease incidence (like Alzheimer's dementia) or populations (in which an enormous and menacing horde of Baby Boomers threatens to tear asunder the very fabric of Western society itself).

- ***The dramatization of resource-sharing across generations, literary generations especially.*** Another thread that stitches my chapters together is how the new suite of concerns raised by population thinking—including resources, scarcity, subsistence, reproduction, and abundance—emerge not just as a plot point in stories about generational difference, or as ways of thinking about the relationship of the present to the past and future, but as a framework for recounting literary-historical modes of inheritance as well. I am especially interested in how the images and thematics of human aging help articulate new insights into the relationship between Romanticism and Victorianism as literary-historical periods. Each chapter therefore examines how the profoundly human temporalities of literary writing—its networks, kinship and familial ties, and positioning with respect to the past and writing yet to come—signal just how embedded the matters of age, aging, and older age are in the imagination of nineteenth-century writers and the legacy of their authorship.

If "[a]esthetics is born as a discourse of the body," as Terry Eagleton writes (75), then we are wise to look to nineteenth-century British writing for signs of a once-new aesthetics of human aging. But why should a book like this matter now? At a moment when the knowledge-producing value of literature and the arts is regularly subordinated to the authority of other disciplinary knowledges, I turn to Ottmar Ette's defense of the literary imagination. "Literature is always ahead of everything else . . . literature has available for its readers areas of knowledge and questions that academic scholarship would have to labor long and hard to bring to life" (Ette 990). My purpose is to make use of ninteenth-century British writing—its insights, yes, but its privileges, limits, prejudices, and colonial legacies too—to reconceptualize the discursive aesthetics of age, aging, and older age, in the present: a time when, in spite of the vast variations that meaningfully particularize age experience, the fact of living in time makes aging an enigmatically universalizing phenomenon. Recent reports from organizations like the United Nations, World Health Organization, National Institutes of Health (US) and World Bank conclude that despite critical axes of difference like gender, race, nationality, class, ability, or sexuality, at this point in the twenty-first century the graying of society constitutes a nearly global demographic phenomenon.[15] Although the aesthetics of aging are necessarily shaped by specificities of national borders and cultural traditions, today the lineaments of ageism, particularly with respect to prejudicial treatment of older persons and aging populations, are disturbingly transnational. As I discuss in the conclusion to this book, the extent to which nineteenth-century British global networks also exported imperial narratives of aging and ageism may only turn out to be fully legible in the present.

As the title of my book indicates, I am drawn to the term "senescence" for how it invokes the evocative interdisciplinary life-course of growing older. Today it is primarily used in reference to the limits of cellular mitosis or division; the Hayflick limit, named after the American anatomist Leonard Hayflick in 1961, demonstrates that in ideal conditions normal human cell populations will divide between 40 and 60 times before dying (one notable exception to this phenomenon are cancer cells, which avoid replicative senescence to become "immortal"). Earlier practice makes use of "senescence" more broadly. The *Oxford English Dictionary* records its first usage in Thomas Blount's *Glossographia* (1656); two and a half centuries later, in an 1894 letter, Robert Louis Stevenson feared "get[ting] a little stale, and my work will begin to senesce." Likewise George Bernard Shaw, who lamented that he was "not adolescing but senescing" in a letter dated 22 June 1909 (thirteen years in advance of G. Stanley Hall's major English-language tome, *Senescence: The Last Half of Life* [1922]). To consider the aesthetics of senescence, then, is to recognize that aging has always invoked the power of contradiction, paradox, and paradoxical thinking: be it of art and science, fact and myth, young and old, self and other. As each chapter of my book demonstrates, the novel becomes a key resource for exploring the implications of increasingly medicalized claims about human nature and the body. Crucially, the speculative power of fiction clears a space to accommodate the realities of paradox and paradoxical thinking: one way of explaining why authors and audiences then, as now, could entertain potentially contradictory arguments in the conceptualization of aging.

In *On Human Longevity, and the Amount of Life Upon the Globe* (1855), the French physiologist Pierre Flourens recalls that Luigi Cornaro, a sixteenth-century Venetian nobleman, attributed his long life (ninety-eight years) to "the gentlest exercises of the mind and heart—literature and benevolence" (6). Cornaro proposes a rather flattering instance of literature's productive interweaving with the aging process but, in the context of this book, such wisdom is particularly suggestive. To narrate is to recount: an intriguing linkage to keep in mind at a moment in history when the birth of demography prioritizes the counting and re-counting of human life. At the dawn of the nineteenth century, the linear progression of maturation is no longer the requisite or *de facto* narrative means of representing life-course. Despite the prevalence of narrative approaches to aging by Age Studies critics (and, of course, the obvious ways that age identities are constructed as narratives, as Swinnen and Port argue [12]), as we shall see, the temporal complexity of the novel becomes an especially productive space for plotting new textualizations of older age as a fluid, non-teleological, and increasingly medicalized state of life: one in which the finitude of individual lifespan often exists in strained reciprocity with the perpetual succession of species. Although this is not necessarily a celebratory or emancipatory view, it does signal the reconceptualization of lifespan that emerged in the wake of the Godwin-Malthus debate.

Nineteenth-century British literature is both entangled with our present intellectual and creative modes and detached from them; for this reason, it can demonstrate why humanistic modes of inquiry continue to matter in our own time. Yet the purpose of this book is not merely to fill in the blanks of our knowledge of aging as a topic of either nineteenth-century British or contemporary Western cultural concern more broadly. It is to consider more widely how an Age Studies perspective might be brought to bear on all-too-familiar concerns about today's "crisis" of the humanities—which frequently manifests as a suspicion that even the habit of reading (never mind conventional modes of literary scholarship) has become, like Wordsworth's ancient leech-gatherer, the near-extinct relic of a bygone past. This book's interest in the thematics of aging means risking the conceptual leaps demanded by multi-disciplinary modes of synthesis; yet my sense is that these are precisely the kind of new conversations that literary scholarship must be prepared to have to realize its longevity. In this respect I take up the challenge of what recent Victorian literature scholars have collectively termed "strategic presentism," which grapples with the thorny matter of *relevance* in literary and humanities scholarship more generally. For all its focus on the long nineteenth century, this book offers an eclectic assessment of why aging and older age are necessary to think about when we consider form, content, history, and the value of the humanities today, especially for readers not fully predisposed to caring about aging or the aesthetic concerns it raises—because by picking up a book we are directly implicated in a public debate about what it means to grapple with imminent obsolescence. By continuing to read, we may already have some sense of why the matter of aging remains of perpetual value to the imagination—literary or otherwise.

Chapter 1 maps an intriguing example of pre- and post-Malthusian literary writing by detailing William Godwin's revolution in thinking about the meaning of aging in his philosophical and literary writing at the turn of the eighteenth century. Chapter 2 explores the strongest reactions to the hostile scepticism of youth (embodied by figures like Malthus and Burke) in a range of "second-generation" Romantic writers, for whom youth becomes not only a prevalent personal and aesthetic branding strategy, but also a disturbing political gambit manifest in the Romantic iconography of fearsome children and geronticide (i.e., elder murder). Against this prevailing idealization of youth, I read Mary Shelley's novels, *The Last Man* (1826) especially, as engaged in a pointed critique of youth's gendered, classed, and reproductive ideology—an instance of what I call "frail Romanticism," which, among other characteristics, serves to critique the surprisingly conservative politics at the heart of the Romantic youth model. In Shelley's case, the personal is crucially related to the political. Where her husband (Percy Bysshe Shelley) and father (William Godwin) were intensely agitated by the apparent incommensurability of youth and age, her own fiction enacts a counterstrategy of disciplinary and generational *rapprochement*: a tactic that expresses some hope for healing the conflict within her familial circle and the concentric age-based anxieties of this literary period.

Chapter 3 further challenges the longstanding wisdom that the Victorian succession of Romanticism reflects the displacement of adolescence by older age, by demonstrating the Victorians' profound interest in the complex linkages of youth and age—specifically through the evocative mid-century interest in physiological "waste" and its counterpart, "repair." I take as my case study the shared premises of George Henry Lewes's medical treatise *The Physiology of Common Life* (1859–60) and George Eliot's novel *Silas Marner: The Weaver of Raveloe* (1861), each of which, in its way, envisions the human body as a lifelong composite of the physiological forces associated with youth and older age. Where Lewes considers the physiological concurrence of waste and repair within the individual, however, Eliot's novel tests and transmutes this simultaneity into the social milieu of human relations. By identifying the ways that growth and decay are fused, I argue that Eliot's multifarious conceptualization of human aging—through her characters, key images, and her own authorial relationship to the literary afterlife of Romanticism—provides the literary-historical imagination with a new apprehension of the aging nineteenth century itself.

Flipping Eliot's happy synthesis on its head, chapter 4 considers how the late Victorians effectively took aging to its extreme by viewing culture itself in the pathologized terms of senility. I focus on the changing coordinates of gender introduced by the "Woman Question" catalyzed by the apparent demographic reality of increasing numbers of unmarried, and often non-reproductive, female bodies: lives that became the hallmark of a pathologically exhausted—and only partially metaphorical—"senile" culture. I read George Gissing's *The Odd Women* (1893) as one response to a new quantification of human aging, a discourse with the capacity to inform, and more often deform, the value of women's life-course especially. On its own and as an exemplar of a "senile topography" evident elsewhere in British literary writing, *The Odd Women* serves as an inceptive synthesis of the literary, medical, and broader cultural tendencies that yoked together major debates concerning massified lives and the biopolitics of aging. I conclude with a discussion of how such representations of youthful senility—and the ironic, queered vision of progress they help chart—mark the radical apogee of the nineteenth century's biopoliticization of gender, longevity, and narratives of growing old, in human as well as national literary timelines.

My conclusion traces the re-emergence, anticipated in part by Anthony Trollope's under-read speculative fiction novel *The Fixed Period* (1882), of a recognizably neo-Godwinian idealism and Malthusian realism in twenty-first-century writings concerning the impact of extended lifespan on the ontological nature of the human subject. Just as Malthus sought to dissolve wildly idealist hopes for immortal life—and in so doing, catalyzed at least one century's literary responses that engaged those terms of debate—so have more recent reconsiderations of what it is to grow old become fertile material for contemporary literary experiments. I close by considering how the transformation of aging (and the distinctly nineteenth-century species of dread that older age has come to provoke) makes new demands on readers and writers for whom aging populations are once again a spur to literary production.

Abbreviations

BE	Catherine Gallagher, *The Body Economic*
CC	Charles Dickens, *A Christmas Carol*
DD	George Eliot, *Daniel Deronda*
DTD	Margaret Gullette, *Declining to Decline*
ELL	George Eliot, *Life and Letters*
F	Mary Shelley, *Frankenstein*
LM	Mary Shelley, *The Last Man*
MM	George Eliot, *Middlemarch*
OED	*Oxford English Dictionary*
PJ	William Godwin, *Enquiry Concerning Political Justice*
SL	William Godwin, *St. Leon: A Tale of the Sixteenth Century*
SLL	Mary Shelley, *Life and Letters*
SM	George Eliot, *Silas Marner*
Z	Erasmus Darwin, *Zoonomia*

Chapter 1

William Godwin and the Artifice of Immortality

In Godwin's *St. Leon: A Tale of the Sixteenth Century* (1799), the immortal protagonist escapes from the Inquisition prison where he was incarcerated for the past twelve years. Having been unable to procure the alchemical apparatus required to make the elixir that would restore his youth, Count Reginald de St. Leon is horrified by both his changed appearance and what it seems to indicate of his mental state. Taking in his own reflection, he describes:

> I found my hair as white as snow, and my face ploughed with a thousand furrows. I was now fifty-four, an age which, with moderate exercise and a vigorous constitution, often appears like the prime of human existence; but whoever had looked upon me in my present condition, would not have hesitated to affirm that I had reached the eightieth year of my age. I examined with dispassionate remark the state of my intellect: I was persuaded that it had subsided into childishness. My mind had been as much cribbed and immured as my body. I was the mere shadow of a man, of no more power and worth than that which a magic lantern produces on a wall. (*SL* 341)

The mirror reflects his new senescence as a curiously thatched composite of images at once realistic and romantic, observed and imagined. For all St. Leon's empiricist resolve, illustrated in comments such as "I found" and "I was persuaded," he unwittingly slips between the mirror of material certainty and the "magic lantern" of imagination. He observes the physiological signs of old age (white hair, wrinkled skin), and immediately describes them figuratively with terrestrial metaphors of "snow" and "ploughed furrows." St. Leon then mentions the fact of his chronological age ("I was now fifty-four")—only to swerve from the first-person observing eye toward the viewpoint of a diffused conjectural onlooker signaled by the compound pronoun "whoever." In terms of his intellect St. Leon feels spectral, a ghost of his former self; in a gesture toward Plato's allegory of the cave, the aged figure in the mirror appears but "the mere shadow of a man." This confusion of real and imagined states is emphasized by the untimely combination of senescence and juvenescence that St. Leon senses in his reflections: both the decrepit body and the childish mind are confined to, and defined by, the crib. Like the cell in which St. Leon finds himself, the body is a troubling site of incarceration. Forced to submit to the arbitrary authority of his Inquisitorial oppressors and, without his alchemical apparatus, to the treacherous insinuations of time as well, St. Leon is obliged to endure a compounded immurement: he is a prisoner both of law and lifespan.

This brief excerpt is emblematic of Godwin's effort to represent senescence in his philosophical as well as his literary writing. In fact, the *Enquiry Concerning Political Justice* (1793, 1796, 1798) and *St. Leon* each foreground—albeit from divergent epistemological perspectives—the related matters of aging, old age, and prolonged life. As described in my introduction, it was Godwin's comments on these topics at the end of *Political Justice* that prompted Malthus to publish his *Essay on the Principle of Population* in 1798. The Godwin-Malthus debate crystallized the terms of a fierce competition staged in the first decades of the nineteenth century between the ideal of human perfectibility and the opposing pressure of population—between, essentially, the imagined romance of immortality and the observed reality of dwindling food supplies. The fact that *St. Leon* was published in 1799—the year following Malthus's scathing rebuttal of the ideas about longevity that were at the heart of both Godwin's treatise and his novel—makes Godwin's work a compelling starting point for apprehending the elusive silhouette of aging and old age in the early years of the nineteenth century.

Like Godwin's enormously successful first novel, *Things as They Are; or, The Adventures of Caleb Williams* (1794), *St. Leon* is widely regarded as a fictionalization of the moral philosophy he articulated in *Political Justice*.[1] Yet little critical attention has been paid to the aspects of *Political Justice* that most directly manifest its intellectual link to *St. Leon*. In a curious concluding section entitled "Of Health, and the Prolongation of Human Life," Godwin asserts that the possibility of a morally perfectible society necessarily implies the potential for considerably prolonged (if not immortal) life.[2] Moreover, despite a rather singular penchant for revising his own arguments, throughout the three editions of *Political Justice* Godwin remains committed to the unlikely hypothesis that life lived according to the principles of political justice "may contribute to prolong our vigour, if not to immortalize it" (*PJ* 2:526). Readers may well pause at such claims. The elimination of old age? The possibility—even if only conjectural—of eternal life? What are we to make of these speculations, especially in light of Godwin's subsequent fictional portrayal of the erasure of old age?

My answer is that *Political Justice* and *St. Leon* together attest to a major shift in Godwin's thinking about the meaning of aging. This shift further registers an acute transitional moment between late-Enlightenment thought and incipient Romanticism, specifically concerning how the aged body is seen to figure the very limits of the human in social discourse. In *Political Justice*, Godwin's anarchist formulation of radically prolonged lifespan is consistent with ideals of individual liberty: just as we ought to seek liberation from the arbitrary shackles of government, so we ought to liberate ourselves from the physiological constraints of lifespan. But rather than portraying the elimination of old age in a utopian manner consistent with those visions, *St. Leon* depicts the destructive consequences of immortality within the context of population. By systematically imagining the lived experience of an immortal life, *St. Leon* reflects ironically on the author's idealist excesses of *Political Justice,* particularly "Of Health," thereby providing an important (if as yet critically neglected) critique of the latter's Enlightenment agenda. *St. Leon* should therefore be understood as a significant revision to Godwin's paean to immortality in *Political Justice*, employing as it does the formal, generic, and intellectual resources of fiction to assert the necessity of individual decline to the collective perpetuity of human life.

In this chapter, I first examine Godwin's portrait of aging in "Of Health," which represents human lifespan as limited, limiting, and incarceral. While *Political Justice* is often read as a response to the political climate of 1790s British radicalism, the chapter's second section revises and supplements this now-familiar context. I focus my discussion on Godwin's logic of speculation in light of similar strategies employed by other contemporary medicalizing discourses that assessed—and, often, imagined possible alternatives to—the inexorability of bodily decline. Taking into account the generic differences evinced by Godwin's speculative philosophical and literary investigations of old age, the final section of this chapter reads *St. Leon* as a radical deviation from *Political Justice*—one that fictionalizes a new biopolitics of lifespan, and gives literary critics new ways to conceptualize both old age and the narrative forms deployed to represent it.

Political Justice and the Aging Body

Godwin's *Enquiry Concerning Political Justice, and its Influence on General Virtue and Happiness* unrelentingly critiques the extensive "insinuat[ion]" of government "into our most secret retirements" (*PJ* 1:4). In each of its editions, Godwin names myriad injuries induced by political institutions including private property, censorship, and customary behaviors such as marriage. If society could only "annihilate the quackery of government," Godwin assures his readers, "the most homebred understanding might be strong enough to detect the artifices of the state juggler that would mislead him" (*PJ* 2:208). Freed from the contorting effects of authoritarian rule, the rational moral virtue intrinsic to all individuals would, over time, grow toward a state of collective perfection; the primary symptom of this would be—among other endowments—the eradication of bodily decline. As Siobhan Ni Chonaill has argued, Godwin's speculations concerning human immortality mark the apogee of his commitment to the utopian idealism reflected more broadly in Britain's Jacobin climate in the last decade of the eighteenth century.[3]

Following its publication in 1793, *Political Justice* received mostly sympathetic reviews, even from critics ideologically opposed to Godwin's ideas (Graham 54). *The Monthly Review* praised *Political Justice* as a "bold and original work" (Graham 72). Others felt obliged to hedge their enthusiasm: *The Literary Magazine and British Review* praised the "many excellent chapters on various subjects of political economy," but felt that these were "interspersed with much extraneous and metaphysical matter" (Graham 70). The 1796 and 1798 revisions of *Political Justice* ranged from minor changes in wording to significant shifts in the implications of Godwin's moral philosophy.[4] The most significant modifications to "Of Health" were his excision of several statements claiming the gradual elimination of the need for sleep (1796), and its formal separation from chapter IX (1798).[5] Godwin also adjusted the scope of his earlier speculations from his 1793 assertion, "If this [question concerning health and longevity] do[es] not lead us to the true remedy [of political justice], it does not follow that there is no remedy. The great object of inquiry will still remain open, however defective may be the suggestions," to the final "If it be false, it leaves the system to which it is appended, in all sound reason, as impregnable as ever" (*PJ* 2:519). Despite his perpetual revisions between 1793 and 1798—which eliminated the "absurd and precipitate judgements" of which he later felt "profoundly ashamed" (Paul 295)—Godwin's conjectures concerning the possibility of defying physiological decline and old age remained constant.

In spite of Romanticism's longstanding associations with the "something beyond the present and tangible" (to borrow Percy Bysshe Shelley's formulation), Godwin's intellectual circle was actively conversant with newly materialist approaches in medicine and science (as work by Alan Richardson, Paul Youngquist, and Neil Vickers has shown). Godwin's own political, fictional, and biographical writings published prior to 1798 (namely *Political Justice, Caleb Williams, The Enquirer*, and the biographical memoir of his late wife, Mary Wollstonecraft, following her sudden death from septicemia in 1797), "evidence both his interest in and familiarity with contemporary science" (Monsam 110). Even in *Political Justice*, his association of maladies in the human body with those of the body politic informs the apparently bizarre premise of radical life extension put forward in "Of Health." Understanding this considerably enriches the intellectual context of *St. Leon*, his most sustained fictional engagement with the question of aging and longevity. In these philosophical and literary assessments of the fate of the body, Godwin emerges both as a late child of British radical dissent and as a father figure—rapidly, if perhaps unknowingly, aging himself—of the Romantic "medical imagination" (Ford 27).

Throughout *Political Justice*, Godwin tellingly collapses the singular and plural meanings of the body, starting with references to "man or body of men" (*PJ* 1:221) or equivalent permutations like "one individual or a body of individuals" (*PJ* 2:3). Frances Ferguson describes Godwin's covertly masculine subject as a problematic model of (a)social being, a "model of a self that must expand infinitely to become identical with the full population of the society, while also remaining untouched by the presence of other consciousnesses" (125). Unsurprisingly, this perfectly systematized ecology of rational bodies struggles to harmonize with human physiology. Consider Godwin's claim that as humanity approaches a state of perfection, the impulse to reproduce will eventually diminish; or that in an ideal society "the whole will be a people of men, and not of children" (*PJ* 2:528). No sex, age, or appetites: *Political Justice* copes with the abstracted materiality of "a people" only by wresting bodies into accordance with the empyrean principles of political justice.

These ideas reach their climax in "Of Health," which begins with "the sublime conjecture" of Benjamin Franklin that "mind will one day become omnipotent over matter":

> But, if the power of intellect can be established over all other matter, are we not inevitably led to ask, why not over the matter of our own bodies? If over matter at however great a distance, why not over matter which, ignorant as we may be of the tie that connects it with the thinking principle, we seem always to carry about with us, and which is our medium of communication with the external universe? (*PJ* 2:519–520)

By turning to the *matter* of "our own bodies," Godwin invokes the spirit of other eighteenth-century writers such as Daniel Defoe, Samuel Richardson, Tobias George Smollett, and Laurence Sterne. As Carol Houlihan Flynn has observed, these authors routinely depicted "the dilemma of the spirit contained by matter that will inevitably betray" (151). Here Godwin is working within a similar paradigm. Repeating the term "matter" four times, he draws attention to the body as a substantial entity but also (and perhaps primarily) a subject for intellectual examination. The *Oxford English Dictionary* lists a wide range of meanings for "matter" in Godwin's time, ranging from its usage as "material for expression; fact or thought as material for a book, speech" to "that which has mass and occupies space; physical substance as distinct from spirit, mind, qualities, actions" and even "physical material of any kind (including blood and other bodily fluids), esp. when only vaguely or generally characterized." By turning to the *matter* of "our own bodies," Godwin invokes—perhaps even puns upon—the lexical ambiguity of this term. In *Political Justice*, normative embodiment demands that individuals behave like expressions of physical matter, and be subject to its laws. Importantly, Godwin's use of the first-person plural (*our* own bodies, ignorant as *we* may be) reiterates this synecdochical coincidence of the subject, expressed both as individual and plural: in the state of political justice, we are at once individualized material and abstracted universal matter.

Godwin's irritation with the bodily accessory is anticipated by the reductionism often associated with Enlightenment conceptions of the body as a mechanical instrument—or, to invoke Julien Offray de La Mettrie's enduring phrase, the *homme-machine*. In fact, Godwin's subjugation of the body to the thinking principle echoes Descartes' famous dictum in book VI of the *Discourse on Method*: "This 'I' by which I am what I am is entirely distinct from the body and could exist without it" (33; I use John Cottingham's English translation here [10])—or, as Descartes writes in *The Passions of the Soul*, that "it is to the body alone that we should attribute everything that can be observed in us to oppose our reason" (346). The mortal coil certainly weighs heavily on the aspirations of *Political Justice*. In the passage above, the mind is obliged to "carry about" the body; it is not simply connected, but "tied." Yet for all his emphasis on the intellectual capabilities, Godwin stops short of portraying the perfected human being as a merely a kind of cerebral avatar (although one might wonder if, in moments of private reverie, he ever dreamed of the immortal and sexless "heads—merely heads" portrayed a century later in H.G. Wells's 1897 *The War of the Worlds* [Wells 149]). Instead, Godwin diverges from Descartes' subjugation of corporeal matter in his concession—however problematic and reluctant it may be—to the bodily "medium" at the basis of political society. Importantly, Godwin's concept of the "mind-limited body" (Ferguson 124) differs from the Enlightenment analogies of perpetual clocks or fountains by its capacity for voluntary action—that is, the mindful and willing application of self to the progression of political justice. Throughout *Political Justice*, and most acutely in "Of Health," the body impedes (even as it enables) the activity of the mind by striving to thwart the "material automatism" of political "tyranny" (*PJ* 1:400).

The matter of the body therefore directs the vocabulary Godwin uses to depict the condition of aging, older age especially, in "Of Health." Beginning with Godwin's recognition of the potentially pathological influence of the mind over corporeal matter, bodily decline quite literally represents the toppling of the physical, psychological, and ethical states he associates with the upward teleology of political justice. When reason resigns itself to vacancy, and benevolence to melancholy, "our external frame *falls* into disorder" (*PJ* 2:522, emphasis added); and "Every time the mind is invaded with anguish and gloom, the frame becomes disordered. Every time langour and indifference creep upon us, our functions *fall* into decay" (*PJ* 2:526, emphasis added). Godwin's formulation of old age in *Political Justice* is indubitably saturated with what more recently would be identified as ageist distain. In so doing, aging in Godwin's "Of Health" evokes what Alan Bewell has called "ideopathology," that is, a malady located "in the sphere of ideas, in human ignorance" as opposed to nature, physiology, or geography (*Colonial Disease* 207). "For writers such as Godwin, Condorcet, and Canis," Bewell writes, "the philosopher is a social physician who uses knowledge and inquiry to cure social and bodily ills. Disease is less a product of nature than a social problem" (207). What interests me about *Political Justice* is its identification of the senilized body as the prime manifestation of social dis-ease, wherein the temporal nature of the body is read as a cipher of political discourse. As the bodily medium surrenders to the corruptive influence of external circumstances, the frame crumbles, before descending freely into earthbound decay.

Political Justice therefore articulates an explicitly gravitational phenomenology of aging, wherein bodily decrepitude becomes a fleshly index of one's falling into age (as Godwin's contemporary idiom would have it). Not only the body, but the mind, is prone to sag and wrinkle. These senilizing effects of gravity—brought on by enforced states of rest, physical immobility, and intellectual stagnation—run contrary to the eighteenth-century compulsion to "run, jump, and swing out of matter" (Flynn 151) that aligns with the conceptual buoyancy of political justice. Godwin thus describes "the aged" as "generally cold and indifferent; nothing interests their attention, or rouses their sluggishness." He speaks of "the approach of inanity and listlessness," and how "a deathlike apathy invades us" (*PJ* 2:523). Devoid of energetic thought, "the aged" come to resemble creeping insects, slug-like, indisposed to action, only barely animated by the deteriorating energy of apathy.

Such decrepitude results from the exertion of gravity on the thinking principle: as if the mind, mechanistically inclined as it may be, must still submit to the same laws that govern the external universe. "How should it be otherwise?" (*PJ* 2:523) Godwin's sigh translates the weight of years into a burdensome bodily thought, as if to literalize Albany's lament from *King Lear*: that "the oldest hath borne most," and "the weight of this sad time we must obey" (5.3.392–394). While Godwin evidently accepts the fact that the body is necessarily subject to physical constraints (nowhere in *Political Justice* does he speak of the potential for human flight, for instance), "Of Health" begs its reader to resist the insinuation of physical laws, particularly gravity, into the activity of the human mind.

In place of the Enlightenment view of the *homme-machine* powered by the internal fire of the heart, Godwin instead posits the mind as the body's perpetual engine. *Political Justice* thus conceives of the healthy individual as an everlastingly youthful organism whose unceasingly active mind-body is primed to resist the entropy and friction implied by older age. Godwin's ideopathology of aging thus specifically targets the Newtonian baggage of matter by arguing that the body is as subject to the weightiness of gravity as it is to the heavy hand of society and the law. A number of his near-contemporaries seem to share such assumptions—indeed, proto-Romantic ideas of the contrary states of innocence and experience appear closely linked to the aesthetics of youth and age articulated in *Political Justice*. Little wonder, then, that the Blakean figures of conventional law are superannuated almost without exception: think of Urizen, the "grey-headed beadles" of "Holy Thursday," and "Aged Ignorance" of *The Gates of Paradise* or *Europe: A Prophecy* (see figure 1.1). Think too of the stifling austerity of Prudence—that "rich,

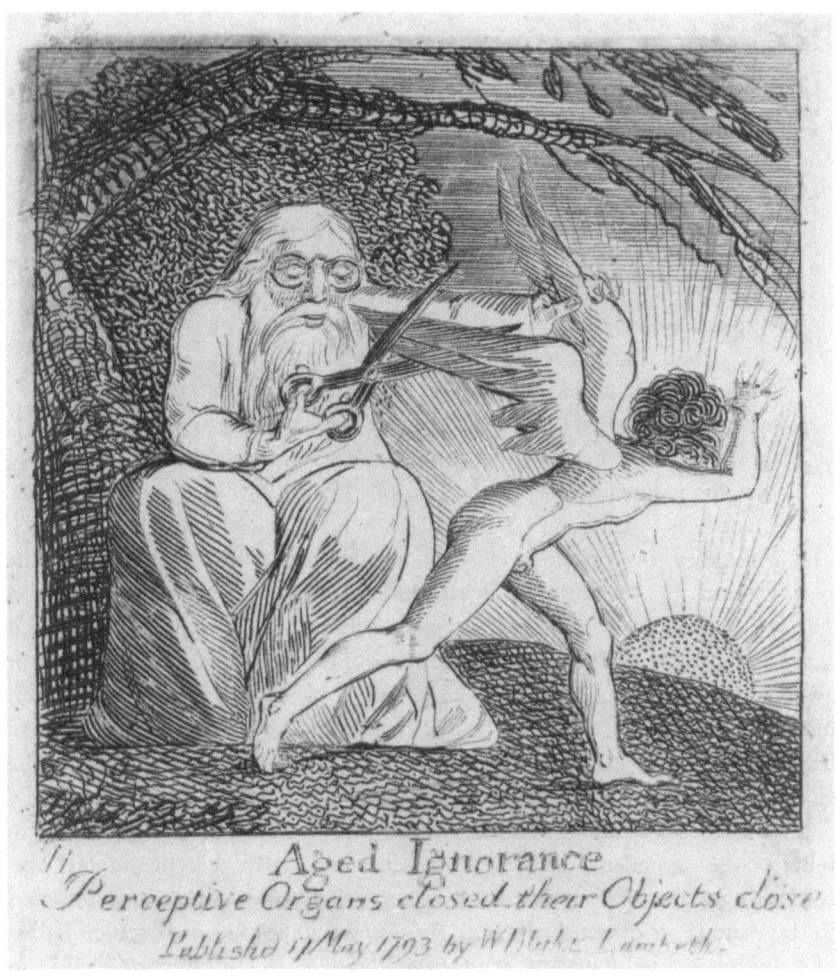

Figure 1.1. William Blake. "Aged Ignorance." From *For the Sexes: The Gates of Paradise*. London, 1793. © The Trustees of the British Museum. All rights reserved.

ugly old maid" described in the *Proverbs of Hell*—that is "courted by Incapacity." For Blake, even nature could be personified in light of such terms:

> Earth rais'd up her head
> From the darkness dread & drear,
> Her light fled:
> Stony dread!
> And her locks cover'd with grey despair. ("Earth's Answer" 1–5,
>   *Songs of Experience*)

We can now see why "Of Health" draws a marked contrast between the buoyancy of youth, and the bondage of age. Youth is associated with affective and physical lightness and motility; its "elasticity" propels it toward ideals of political justice:

> Why is it that a mature man loses that elasticity of limb, which characterises the heedless gaiety of youth? The origin of this appears to be, that he desists from youthful habits. He assumes an air of dignity, incompatible with the lightness of childish sallies. He is visited and vexed with the cares that rise out of our mistaken institutions, and his heart is no longer satisfied and gay. His limbs become stiff, unwieldy and aukward [sic]. This is the forerunner of old age and of death. (*PJ* 2:521)

This passage epitomizes Godwin's gravitational phenomenology of aging. The mature man, by contrast to the youthful one, can enjoy only a deceptive "air" of dignity, contaminated by the falsity "visited" upon him, like an illness or affliction. Those "mistaken institutions" usurp the self, forcing it away from the propulsive energy of political justice. By contrast, the habit of youth is perpetual action. As a result, the temporal character of political justice asserts itself as ethical process of living, one that resists bringing the character of gravity to bear upon daily life.

Rather than taking issue with long life or even aging *per se*, Godwin rebukes the moralized physical traits that habitually accompany old age. Interestingly, the aged constitution is not necessarily diametrically opposed to the conditions of youth. In fact, *Political Justice* implies that settled habits of thinking—a tendency to resist new ideas, to feel most comfortable in intellectual or behavioural "resting places" (*PJ* 1:66)—may in fact occur at any point in the life-course. As Godwin points out, an individual at any age may begin to recognize patterns in worldly phenomena and feel "inclined to abridge the process of deliberation, and act today conformably to the determination of yesterday" (*PJ* 1:65). Such habits of decorum, custom, social conduct, and even language make the voluntary mental practice of "perpetual revisal" (*PJ* 1:69) less likely—thus producing the oppressive stagnation typified for Godwin by the symptoms of older age.

There is a clear parallel here with Romantic ideas of the imagination as a process of defamiliarization and rejuvenation. The language of poets, Percy Shelley writes in "A Defence of Poetry," is "vitally metaphorical . . . if no new poets should arise to create afresh the associations which have been thus disorganized, language will be dead to all the nobler purposes of human intercourse" (747). In its exaltation of perpetual freshness, replenishment, and the new, we might detect here an implicit critique of aging. In the "Defence," Shelley argues that poetry "redeems from decay the visitations of the divinity in man" (759); in "Ode to the West Wind" he similiarly speaks of the "heavy weight of hours" that "has chained and bowed / One too like thee: tameless, and swift, and proud" (*Poetical*; lines 55–56); and in *The Cenci* he presents a brutal, incestuous assault against youthful rebellion. All these almost certainly take their cue from the aesthetics of senescence articulated in *Political Justice*.

Of course, Godwin was not the first to assert that the thinking principle was a factor in the aging process. The eternally aging Struldbrugs in Jonathan Swift's *Gulliver's Travels* (a text Godwin also mentions in *Political Justice*) exhibit the mind's stagnation as a chief symptom—though not the cause—of old age. In this often-cited portion of Swift's satirical travel narrative (written in 1726, amended 1735), Gulliver's Tithonian error is highlighted by presenting a scenario in which prolonged life is realized in the absence of "youth, health, and vigour" (Swift 1024). Significantly, the Struldbrugs' most offensive features are not physical or even intellectual, but behavioral: their propensity to be "opinionative, peevish, covetous, morose, vain, talkative . . . incapable of friendship, and dead to all natural affection"—qualities not associated with any diminishment of their mental powers, but with "the dreadful prospect of never dying" (1025). Gulliver tells us that the best fate for a Struldbrug is to "turn to dotage, and entirely lose their memories; these meet with more pity and assistance, because they want many bad qualities which abound in others" (1025). In contrast to Godwin, Swift hints that the aged may be better off embracing the quiescence of their advanced years, freed from the mental agitation of recollection. Swift's portrayal anticipates aspects of Godwin's position concerning the role of mind in bodily decay. But Godwin's insistence that the mind should be able to assert command—not merely over the body's voluntary actions, but also over its internal processes (such as blood circulation), and even over external physical laws such as gravity and temporality—marks a transitional moment, as Gary Kelly has shown, between Enlightenment idealism and Romantic materialism.[6]

Godwin's incipient Romanticism is also signaled by another innovation in his interpretation of old age. His repugnance for involuntary fixity, for example, is in stark contrast to the generationally figured value placed on custom and predictability by David Hume in his *Enquiry Concerning Human Understanding* (1748). When asked why an aged husbandsman is more skillful than a younger one, Hume claims that "a *certain uniformity* in the operation of the sun, rain, and earth" teaches the "old practitioner . . . the rules by which this operation is governed and directed" (65, emphasis added). Hume describes a seasonal narrative of life-course reflective of the predictable cycling of the stages-of-life model. Despite the common perception that Godwin manifests more Humean tendencies in later editions of *Political Justice,* "Of Health" rejects that static pastoral reliance on knowledge that is effortlessly accumulated, in a sort of passive process of life-long learning.[7]

For Godwin, any loss of will to "live while we live"—that is, to act with deliberate intent in pursuit of a goal, rather than merely for the sake of social decorum or expectations associated with the stages-of-life motif—condemns the mind to corporeal captivity (*PJ* 2:526). Aging, then, must be a voluntary process. If it is not, and truth must "recommence her carreer [sic] every thirty years" with the birth of a new generation (*PJ* 2:528), the temporal nature of the body is a fatal obstacle in the onward march of perfectibility. Unlike Hume, with his nostalgia for the continuity of the past, Godwin takes issue with the customary shackles of biology on human potential.[8] As one contemporary would write in 1807:

> The little Actor cons another part;
> Filling from time to time his "humorous stage"
> With all the Persons, down to palsied Age,
> That Life brings with her in her equipage;
>   As if his whole vocation
>   Were endless imitation.
> (Wordsworth, "Intimations of Immortality from Recollections of Early Childhood," 102–107)

Not unlike William Wordsworth's suspicion here of unthinking habit's "earthly freight"—"And custom lie upon thee with a weight, / heavy as frost, and deep almost as life!" (131–132)—*Political Justice* forcefully asserts that to avoid senescence, one must resist nature's interminable cycling and the dictates, the fiction even, of temporal decline.

Godwin's critique of aging effectively rewrites the Enlightenment ideal of perpetuity as a voluntary condition of the mind. Taken in context, his speculation in "Of Health" ("Is it not then highly probable, in the process of human improvement, that we may finally obtain an empire over every articulation of our frame?" [*PJ* 2:524]) should appear somewhat less absurd than it may at first. In fact, it reveals an important rift at the heart of Godwin's philosophical project. An anecdote (possibly apocryphal) states that after Wordsworth read *Political Justice*, he told another student to "throw aside your books of chemistry, and read Godwin on Necessity."[9] What becomes clear in reading *Political Justice* is that Godwin's speculative solution to the problem of the body in time is to take up agency against the temporalized dictates of necessity itself. By divorcing old age from its association with nature, Godwin introduces a newly politicized meaning of aging. More than this, "Of Health" introduces a significantly altered view of life-course. Senescence is no longer an "age" or "stage" of life, but is itself a state, a physiological symptom of the tyrannical authority of time—identical in effect to the influence of its political counterpart, government.[10] The passage from *St. Leon* I cited at the outset of this chapter illustrates this Godwinian equivalence in *Political Justice:* old age is both a symbol and embodied symptom of one's subjection to the normative laws of politics and temporality. As the Marquis de Damville cautions Reginald de St. Leon, the aging process exerts its own dismal "tyranny" (*SL* 83).

Aging's Speculative Fictions

Needless to say, Godwin's utopian optimism about the possibility of eradicating old age was not universally shared. Shortly after the publication of the first edition of 1793, the *Critical Review* found Godwin's ideas categorically absurd: "The acme . . . of Mr Godwin's speculations, are his extraordinary reasonings concerning the prolongation of human life, even to 'immortality.' Such a hypothesis requires only to be mentioned to be refuted" (Graham 69). Similarly, the *British Critic* lamented—fittingly, in light of the weighty subject matter—that the author "has taken an immeasurable flight, on the waxen wings they [Godwin's major sources: Condorcet, Rousseau, and Helvetius] instructed him to fabricate; and before the conclusion of his book is perfectly in the clouds, to fall, like Icarus" (307–308).

Yet Godwin's influence cannot be overestimated, not only at this time but throughout the nineteenth century—in spite of his own spectacular fall from public favor in the decade following the publication of *Political Justice*. In his indispensable study of Godwin's philosophy, Mark Philp shows that the book "was firmly tied to the language, conventions and arguments he found in his social milieu and that, as a result, much of what he argued was persuasive to the radicals and the intellectuals of the time" (230). With this in mind, I want to reorient and extend the scope of the intellectual context usually associated with Godwin's work by examining the role of speculation in medicalized investigations of old age in the years around 1800.[11] Such reorientation is necessary to address lingering scholarly misconceptions that Godwin was a mere naïve idealist, and to recognize his intellectual position in relation to emergent materialist debates in the Romantic period. To parse Godwin's ideas about the prolongation of life, I now turn to his rhetorical parallels with other speculative assessments of aging at the turn of the century. The speculative mode is essential to constructing and asserting the fictionality of old age, and helps us to understand how Godwin's philosophical speculative strategy ultimately demands a specifically novelistic intervention to correct the error at the basis of his claims in "Of Health."

In the 1790s, Godwin was not alone in his conviction of the need for intellectual approaches to the prolongation of life. Numerous texts circulated widely on the topic of older age: Cicero's *De Senectute*, as well as the writings of Hippocrates, Galen, and Aristotle, had remained authoritative sources throughout the early modern period, tending to view old age as the final stage in life's drama.[12] But as secularism gained traction throughout Enlightenment Europe, the possibility of prolonged life on earth (as opposed to religious figurations of the afterlife) meant that "death need no longer be obligatory, but an optional extra" (Mulvey-Roberts, "Physic" 152). One of the earliest and most enduring responses was the demand for literature depicting extended or immortal life. Such portrayals—for example, of historical figures such as Ponce de León, the early-sixteenth-century Spanish explorer and alleged discoverer of the fountain of youth in Florida, clearly the source for Godwin's titular protagonist—often obscured distinctions between fact and fiction, history and legend.[13]

Such narratives of "prolongevity" (to use Gerald J. Gruman's term) were not limited to the imaginative realm. Practical remedies for extending life involving diet, exercise, and physical hygiene were widely available, as were less credible antidotes peddled by unscrupulous practitioners: transfusions of animal blood, benevolent astrological constellations, and the rejuvenating effects of "effluvia"—the breath of young women. Despite the professionalization of chemistry throughout this period, the possibility of eliminating old age stayed firmly on what Gotthilf Heinrich von Schubert evocatively termed the "night side of the sciences."[14] Even Thomas Beddoes (1760–1808), the politically radical British physician (and like Godwin, a member of the Johnson Dissenting circle), "earned extremes in respect and suspicion" for his investigations into the recuperative effects of oxygen on age-related ailments such as arthritis (Fox). By the time Godwin was writing *Political Justice*, alchemy represented "a subversive agenda" for radicals and reactionaries alike (Mulvey-Roberts, "Physic" 163). As we saw in my introduction, counter-revolutionary fearmongers like Edmund Burke negatively associated alchemy with political, religious, and scientific dissent, while *St. Leon* worked to critique such reactionary discourse by referencing the destruction of Joseph Priestley's chemistry laboratory in the 1796 Birmingham Riots. Although medieval thaumaturges such as Hermippus, Gualdi, and Paracelsus—all historical and imaginative sources for *St. Leon*—were widely regarded with Enlightenment scorn, by the late eighteenth century the secular grail-object of alchemical lore, the *elixir vitae*, remained a popular if ideologically ambiguous cultural motif.

Yet evading senescence could also be viewed as a "legitimate" inquiry. One of the most significant contributions to medicalizing discourses of aging at this time was *The Art of Prolonging Life* (first published in German in 1796, and translated into English in 1797) by the German writer Christoph Wilhelm Hufeland (1762–1836). The personal physician of luminaries such as Kant, Goethe, Schiller, and King Friedrich Wilhelm III, Hufeland proposed a regimen for the maintenance of youthful vigor based on the principle of *Lebenskraft*—"vital power" or "life force."[15] The doctor is unequivocal: almost all natural deaths before the age of one hundred should be considered artificial or premature. Hufeland writes: "we may . . . with the greatest probability, assert, that the organization and vital power of man are able to support a duration and activity of 200 years" (109). Citing anecdotes of cententarians, and demographic data gathered from England and continental Europe, Hufeland asserted that the body's fixed stock of vital power would be dissipated less rapidly by following the Baconian dictum of *modus omnibus in rebus*—moderation in all things—particularly in diet, lifestyle, and temperament. The treatise was immediately successful in Germany, and propelled Hufeland to a kind of celebrity status. Translations (and pirated copies) were soon available throughout Europe. In Britain, *The Art of Prolonging Life* continued to be cited with admiration by medical, lay, and literary commentators for more than a century—although, like Godwin's claims for extended life, Hufeland's were met with a combination of interest and reservation.[16]

While there is no direct evidence to suggest that Godwin read *The Art of Prolonging Life* as he was writing *Political Justice*, Hufeland's text demonstrates noteworthy parallels with the "medical utopianism" of Godwin's treatise ("Futures," Porter 35).[17] Both share a belief in human perfectibility and the possibility of judiciously cultivating both body and mind. Like Godwin, Hufeland asserts that corporeal and intellectual hygiene are twin pursuits essential to "rational being" (107). He writes that "physical and moral health . . . flow from the same sources; become blended together; and when united, the result is HUMAN NATURE ENNOBLED AND RAISED TO PERFECTION" (xii, emphasis in original). In place of political justice, the vital power is drawn from a mainstay of classical medical thought, which held all animal and vegetable life to be animated by a vivifying principle. Remarkable, however, is Hufeland's description of this conjectural biological principle as "the most subtle, the most penetrating, and the most invisible agent of nature" (35) comparable to other accepted but imperceptible physical phenomena such as "light, electricity, and magnetism, to which . . . it seems to have the closest affinity" (35). Although this notion of a limited vital power would likely not appeal to Godwin (smacking as it does of Calvinist predetermination and even, perhaps, the brute mechanism of the *homme-machine*), Hufeland's references to the transcendence of reason over nature, and his suspicion of sleep or states of "apparent death," are certainly reminiscent of Godwin's call to arms against the ideopathology of old age. Most pertinently, when Hufeland argues that the sclerotic "rigidity" (158) of old age might be the effect of "wretched political calculat[ions]" such as slavery and foundling houses (103), we might recall the ossified body described in "Of Health." Though not as explicitly committed to overhauling social conditions as his British contemporary, Hufeland nevertheless flirts with an emergent biopolitics of aging in his desire to account for external circumstances that excessively drain the body of vigor. *The Art of Prolonging Life* proves that neither Godwin's claims concerning the fate of the body nor his approach to the etiology of aging was as idiosyncratic as either might appear today.

The fact that Hufeland's ideas were respected throughout the nineteenth century should prompt us to consider how such medicalized explorations of the causes of old age were linked by their use of imaginative, rather than strictly empirical, strategies. Situating Godwin in this sympathetic intellectual climate permits a richer understanding of how *St. Leon* uses speculation as a species of intellectual intervention into aging.[18] As Peter Stockwell writes, this "imaginative figuring of reality" ideally creates a "material reality of visualization" (6) that allows readers to understand and empathize with the fictional world. Unlike deception, which presents falsehood as truth, speculation intends a productive confusion of the real and the imaginary. By visualizing things that do not actually exist, such conjectures may even serve as proto-empirical supplements to scientific knowledge. In the absence of established theory, writes twentieth-century philosopher of science Karl Popper, there is *"no more rational procedure than the method of trial and error—of conjecture and refutation"* (51, emphasis in original). Speculation attempts to bridge the epistemological gap between things as they are and things as they could, or would, or should be.

Such imaginative strategies link the development of mid-eighteenth-century science with that of the novel. As John Bender has shown, both disciplinary spheres engage in the narrativization of circumstantial evidence and appeal to ostensible probability; while the novel is manifestly fiction, scientific discourse—despite its factuality—could not "fully escape implication in that very fictionality" (18). George-Louis Buffon, the French naturalist and author of the 36-volume *Natural History* (published between 1749 and 1788), exemplifies the appeal of speculative science at that time. By "rejecting fantastic premises . . . and insisting upon exact analysis of observable physical fact," Buffon employs factual observation "to free a space for strictly controlled speculation in the form of hypotheses that answer the question 'how'" (Bender 20). Hufeland may have imagined his invisible "vital principle," but his records, anecdotes, and observations in *The Art of Prolonging Life* seek to explain or at least associate the origins of old age with empirically-determinable phenomena. Moreover—and this becomes increasingly important to the professional study of aging throughout the nineteenth century—Hufeland maintains his epistemological premise of the vital principle without resorting to the "miserable" (138) clandestine practices of the alchemists, whose promises he felt were not just impossible but also destructive. For Godwin and Hufeland, at the very end of the eighteenth century, the study of aging demands a similarly bifocal technique capable of coping with both the facts and fiction of lived experience.

Obviously, speculation is an essential strategy for idealists to use in their predictions, as exemplified by "Of Health." Godwin makes this clear in his opening statement of method: "It may therefore be allowed us, to make use of this occasion, for indulging in certain speculations upon this article. What follows, must be considered, as eminently a deviation into the land of conjecture." Yet he hedges this claim by continuing, "If it be false, it leaves the system to which it is appended, in all sound reason, as impregnable as ever" (*PJ* 2:519). Perhaps most striking is Godwin's suggestion that this section is any more speculative than the other premises articulated elsewhere in *Political Justice*. His choice of words ("indulging," "deviation") acknowledges its potentially corruptive effects upon an otherwise "sound" and indeed "impregnable" body of text. While Godwin, like the proto-empiricist Popper imagines, invites his conjectures to be falsified (perhaps necessarily, given the Gordian snarl of alchemical, medical, philosophical, and literary ideas associated then, as now, with bodily decay), his arguments for the elimination of old age certainly test even the most generous parameters of possibility. From phrases ("it seems," "it appears to be") to point of view (the use of first-person plural pronouns: "we," "our") to more dubious rhetorical flourishes (particularly the forced choice signaled by the interrogative "is this not . . ." and its permutations throughout this section), Godwin's philosophical speculations struggle to stimulate a rationalist identification with the obscured reality of political justice. Godwin's method of extrapolation is unable to register (or unwilling to accommodate) differences between the singular and the plural, individual bodies and the collective, the real and the hypothetical, the present and the future. In effect, the empathetic impulse of speculation is usurped by Godwin's logic of synecdoche. "The whole will be a people of men, and not of children": Godwin's utopian vision is manifestly hostile toward any variation, even that of generation.

Godwin's speculations can thus be said to "radicalize" his philosophy, in a manner consistent with Tilottama Rajan and Julia M. Wright's discussion of "mode" in Romantic writing (4). More than just an adjectival derivative of a statically conceived generic category (e.g., the elegaic mode vs. the genre of elegy), "modes are a mechanism for bringing new material into culture . . . . By expanding literature to engage it with other areas of experience, modes also expand the range of the genre, defined more narrowly as a 'kind' with specific formal features" (4). The speculative mode of *Political Justice* effectively expands the jurisdiction of philosophical discourse into the biopolitics of aging. In so doing, "Of Health" not only writes the body into Godwin's moral-political philosophy (as did Descartes and others long before), but also employs the speculative mode to explain the temporal experience of the body as an ideopathological expression of political tyranny. Between this work and the publication of *St. Leon*, however, Godwin's speculation shifts from a mode of philosophical inquiry toward the literary. The speculations of *Political Justice* become the fictional referent of *St. Leon*.

By now it should be apparent why Godwin's speculations on old age constitute a necessary conclusion to *Political Justice*. First, they demonstrate a certain realism: in Godwin's time the concept of prolonged life was plausible, if highly provisional, as evinced by other works like *The Art of Prolonging Life*. Godwin's ideas effectively resist the "tyranny of the real" (Stockwell's aptly Godwinian phrase, 6) while remaining intellectually moored—however tenuously—to the known parameters of the material world. Second, speculation enables Godwin to account for the visible effects on the aging body of forces whose causal mechanisms exist outside of the empirical realm: what might be referred to today as *social determinants of health* such as education, law, employment, and political conditions. Third, speculative exercise is exactly the kind of intellectual medicine Godwin prescribes for staving off mental and physical decrepitude. (In this regard, he seems almost modern: just as our present anti-aging paradigm encourages diligent application to crosswords, Sudoku puzzles, and the like to keep neural synapses firing, Godwin recognized that the perpetual engine of the youthful mind was best kept in motion by the furiously active pistons of intellectual activity.) The question of bodily finitude therefore invites us to read "Of Health" as "a provocation rather than an endpoint" (Handwerk 82). Indeed, the ideas Godwin expressed in *St. Leon* make this novel an ironic epitaph to his golden half-decade (1793–1798)—and, in fact, to his whole philosophical career.

St. Leon and the Long Life of Species

In her essay "The Rise of Fictionality," Catherine Gallagher argues that the foundational claim of the novel is the distinction made by Henry Fielding's narrator in *Joseph Andrews* (1742), who seeks to describe "not men, but manners; not an individual, but a species." Rather than the allegorical transposition of persons that populated earlier narrative forms, the novel's human referent was a generalization, rather than an embodied extratextual example, of character: "The fictionality defining the novel inhered in the creation of instances, rather than their mere selection, to illustrate a class of persons" ("Fictionality" 342). Gallagher's definition has important implications for how we read *St. Leon*, since the "individual"—conceived according to the synecdochical logic of *Political Justice*—almost ceases to exist as such within the social framework of the novel.

Although primarily concerned with novelistic fictionality, Gallagher's account helps us understand how speculation functions differently in Godwin's philosophical and literary writing. In *St. Leon*, Godwin shifts away from an impersonally philosophical mode of imagining old age to figuring it concretely—thus actively implicating the reader in the novel's fictional world. As Gallagher writes, the reader—unlike the character—"occupies the lofty position of *one who speculates on the action,* entertaining various hypotheses about it." This reaction magnifies the more abstract demand that earlier fiction placed on its readers, which was "*to take the reality of the story itself as a kind of suppositional speculation*" (Gallagher 346, emphasis added). Godwin's second novel is thus an exemplar of Rajan's observation that "[n]ovels are, in effect, a form of speculation" (*Narrative* 158).

The best way to approach Godwin's second novel may be as an example of what in *Political Justice* he calls the "intellectual branch" of medicine. As illustrated in the passage from *St. Leon* that opens this chapter, old age constitutes a strikingly fluid category encompassing disintegrative elements at once realistic and romantic, factual and metaphorical, physiological and imaginary—not unlike the elusive form of the novel itself. Far from merely recycling Godwin's philosophical premises, the fictionality of *St. Leon* works as a corrective to the philosophical speculations in "Of Health." Ultimately, the novel deems old age to be essential to the perpetuation of human life, rather than (as Mulvey-Roberts phrased it) an "optional extra." The fact that *St. Leon* was written as a partial response to Malthus is further indicated by Godwin's explicit praise; in his *Spital Sermon* of 1801, Godwin professes his "unfeigned approbation and respect" for both Malthus's *Essay* "and the spirit in which it is written"—even admitting "some pride, in so far as by my writings I gave the occasion, and furnished an incentive, to producing so valuable a treatise."[19] Thus we misunderstand a key aspect of Godwin's writing and, more generally, the British radicals' interest in immortality, if we disregard discussions of radically prolonged life as merely protracted Enlightenment enthusiasm or ham-fisted gothic kitsch. In this fictional case study of a disastrously unbounded life, *St. Leon* rejects the essentially individualistic ethos of *Political Justice* in favor of associating older age with the very possibility of biological generation and human perfectibility.

A brief summary. Godwin's second novel presents the first-person confessional of Reginald de St. Leon, a young French aristocrat, whose fortunes change drastically against the backdrop of the Protestant Reformation. Despite an admirable upbringing, St. Leon becomes a compulsive gambler, eventually plunging his wife and family into dire poverty. His miserable prospects seem to improve when he is offered the philosopher's stone (which enables the perpetual production of gold) and the *elixir vitae* (which gives immortal life) by the mysterious, superannuated stranger Zampieri. Instead of assisting his benevolent aims, however, the alchemical gift eventually leads to the destruction of his family and, in due course, his exile from all human relations. In addition to Godwin's well-known concession to the importance of the "domestic affections" in its prefatory remarks, *St. Leon* also marks a startling reversal of the views expressed in "Of Health" (*SL* 53).

Yet the novel's opening paragraph seems to recapitulate *Political Justice*'s idealized condition of immortality, as St. Leon wonders—with some cheek on the part of Godwin the novelist—whether we might not subordinate the ideals of political justice to the magnificent endowments of alchemy: "What is political liberty compared with unbounded riches and immortal vigour?" (*SL* 54). Godwin's use of the gothic "apparatus" of alchemy as a plot device illustrates Gary Kelly's claim that the English Jacobins tended to associate such practices with "the eternal ambition of man to transcend himself" (213). In St. Leon, the *elixir vitae* further works to signify the transitional, secularizing, individualist ethos evident in medicalized interests in the prolongation of life during the 1790s. By integrating metaphysical aspirations with the gross corporeality of the body, Godwin's first-person narrative of the immortal personifies the ultimate transgression of the narrative of decline in old age.

St. Leon recollects his elation after realizing the effects of his "julep" (*SL* 349):

> "What!" exclaimed I, "these limbs, this complicated but brittle frame, shall last forever! No disease shall attack it; no pain shall seize it; death shall withhold from it forever his abhorred grasp! Perpetual vigour, perpetual activity, perpetual youth, shall take up their abode with me! Time shall generate in me no decay, shall not add a wrinkle to my brow, or convert a hair of my head to grey!" (*SL* 188)

Behold the *homme-machine*, liberated from the ideopathological connotations of "seiz[ure]"—physical, mechanical, political—described in "Of Health." Like his now-perpetual bodily frame, St. Leon's observations are generated with no dissipation of energy. Yet if we examine his repetitive refrains—"No . . . no . . . no"; "perpetual . . . perpetual . . . perpetual"; the almost metrical regularity of "shall"—the effect is, in fact, one of stasis. In this passage, the mortal condition of old age and the transcendent ideal of immortality remain strangely proximal to each other, locked in a dyad whose terms are separated only by the negative: disease/no disease, pain/no pain, decay/no decay. For all its amplified exclamation, St. Leon's language conspicuously recycles words and speech patterns in a way that calls to mind those "resting places" Godwin once described as anathema to youth (*PJ* 1:65).

However, despite its initial resonances with "Of Health," *St. Leon* ultimately leads readers to consider how eternal individual vigor might thwart the collective goals of a benevolent society. Justine Crump and Marie Mulvey-Roberts have both separately noted that the boons of monetary wealth and immortality constitute socially disruptive economies in the novel. Mulvey-Roberts points out that in close imitation of unbridled wealth, unlimited life upsets the established system of social relations by exerting undue influence on the "invisible hand" of reproduction (*Gothic* 45). And Crump observes that alchemy—together with gambling, St. Leon's earlier vice—are "irregular modes of acquisition that threaten the orderly, visible circulation of capital" (402). Like other critical readings of *St. Leon*, these insights underscore the significance of St. Leon's wealth, effectively relegating his longevity to a thematic afterthought. In many ways this is not surprising. The novel itself seems to assign more weight to the former than the latter in describing alchemy's goal. St. Leon speaks of "these two grand and inseparable branches, the art of multiplying gold, and of defying the inroads of infirmity and death" (*SL* 53), and the text is littered with passages that subordinate the *elixir vitae* to material riches ("Exhaustless wealth, if communicated to all men, would be but an exhaustless heap of pebbles and dust; and nature will not admit her everlasting laws to be so abrogated, as they would be by rendering the whole race of sublunary man immortal" [*SL* 186]).

If, as Crump and others have argued, the problem of St. Leon's wealth is that of disrupted economic circulation, then the truly ruinous consequence of immortality would be its interruption of biological generation and generational succession—an apparent recalibration of the Burkean organic body politic and its politics of inheritance. Readers of Godwin's "graver productions" (to use his own phrasing in the novel's preface) might not expect to find that in *St. Leon*, immortality would eventually induce the very rigidity and stasis associated with old age described in "Of Health." At one point the protagonist describes himself as standing "in the middle point, like one of those invincible repulsive powers hid in the storehouse of nature" (*SL* 440), like an embodiment of Hufeland's fascination with similarly invisible forces, like magnetism, on vital life. The mere prospect of radically prolonged life collapses past and future into an interminably lived present, disrupting the succession of the old by the young demanded by generation: "Months, years, cycles, centuries! To me these are but as indivisible moments. I shall never become old" (*SL* 188).

Even before meeting the aged alchemist Zampieri, St. Leon has a relentless attachment to the tastes and attitudes of youth. His character resists generationally figured roles; he often describes himself in childish terms: "my infant mind" (*SL* 206); "puerile eagerness" (*SL* 260); "a mere tyro" (*SL* 304); and his behavior, especially prior to receiving the elixir, might best be described as insufferably adolescent. In the early days of their marriage, Marguerite tries to extract St. Leon from his "infantine taste for magnificence and expense" and quite literally make an honest man of him (*SL* 120). Despite several crises and resolutions, however, he refuses to act the part of a mature man—first, by way of his behavior, and secondly, by means of the body itself, as the elixir brings St. Leon face-to-face with eternal youth.

Anne Chandler has discussed St. Leon's stubbornly adolescent tendencies in light of Rousseau's portrayal of pubescent male self-fashioning in *Emile*, noting that the novel's "odd emphasis on ironies of age-based *mis*recognition" effectively scrambles "the assumed age differential, and with it the signals of normative age" (406). Yet St. Leon's juvenile attachments are, in fact, a symptom of the novel's deeper concern with his disruption of generational succession. In an important scene that foreshadows the novel's concerns with aging and generation, St. Leon is struck by a mysterious illness and dutifully attended to by his son, Charles, who with his three younger sisters give up their food so that their father might eat. Godwin's far-fetched portrait of famished yet morally composed toddlers is underlined by the contrast he draws between the children's stoicism and St. Leon's frantic outburst. He compares himself to Ugolino, the historical figure immortalized in Dante's *Inferno*, whose sons offered him their bodies to eat as they starved together in prison:

> We are perishing by inches. We have not provision for the coming day! No, no; something desperate, something yet unthought of, must be attempted! I will not sit inactive, and see my offspring around me die in succession. No, by Heaven! Though I am starving like Ugolino, I am not, like Ugolino, shut up in a dungeon! The world is open; its scenes are wide; the resources it offers are, to the bold and despairing, innumerable! I am a father, and will show myself worthy of the name! (*SL* 147)

In this moment of personal and intertextual epiphany, St. Leon realizes—at last—how much his offspring are dependent upon him. He perceives the likeness of his situation to Ugolino's, but also the difference. *He* is not condemned to allegorical or synecdochal repetition of that class of desperate persons who would cannibalize the forward motion of generational succession: the world, like his momentary affiliation with Ugolino, is "open" to variation from type.[20] The developmental conventions of the *Bildungsroman* demand that the individual develop in response to their situation, and St. Leon's change is a drastic one. With "little more than the strength of a new born child" (*SL* 150), he shakes off his pathologically adolescent state to assert his mature role of fatherhood—a grown man with the capacity to act and resist repeating the narratives of the literary past. At this crucial moment in the novel, Reginald's fictional logic—though "I am like Ugolino, I am not Ugolino"—helps him take up the conceptual category and "worthy . . . name" of "father" over "traitor." St. Leon defines himself anew by type, by manner, and, most significantly, by his relationship to an expressly biologically figured notion of species.

After this incident, six years of "peace and tranquillity" (*SL* 155) pass before St. Leon—out of a distorted sense of necessity, both for himself and for his family—accepts Zampieri's accursed alchemical "gift." (Presumably Godwin designed this hiatus in order to allow Reginald's small children to grow old enough to make the next phase of the plot credible.) Despite his prior conviction that he will escape Ugolino's fate, the transformation does not augur well. Just moments after his elated recognition of his own immortality, St. Leon glimpses how alchemy works to dismantle the connection between domesticity and biological being, a man and "the race of mankind"—both of which now appear "insignificant" to him: "I felt a degree of uneasiness at the immeasurable distance that was put between me and the rest of my species. I found myself alone in the world" (*SL* 188). Increasingly estranged from his wife, Marguerite, and his children ("they were now . . . nothing to me" [*SL* 189]), St. Leon finds it difficult to concern himself with the mortal needs of mere "ephemeron" (*SL* 189); employing another unsettling entomological metaphor, Godwin's immortal protagonist describes how he "can form no true and real attachment to the insect of an hour" (*SL* 298).

Godwin's novel displaces St. Leon from exactly the social human relations that call out for political justice. *St. Leon*'s ostensible narrative of development is therefore a perverse one: St. Leon begins to repeat (without reflection or acknowledgment) the same injurious adolescent behaviors of the past, thereby divorcing age from its traditional connotations with maturity and cumulative understanding (what Fredric Jameson has termed "the ideology of experience" [*Archaeologies* 337]). Unlimited lifespan critically undermines the *Bildungs*-narrative structure, which assumes a gradual progress of maturation if not perfectibility.

St. Leon's perpetual failures imply that perfectibility necessarily depends on the aging process. His travesty of generational succession is manifested in the unfortunate fates of his daughters especially (Charles has long since disowned his father, left his family, and joined the army). Following the death of Marguerite—on her deathbed it is unclear whether she hopes or demands that St. Leon "burst [his] fetters and be free" of his offspring—he returns, apparently disguised by youth, to present his daughters with (counterfeited) evidence that their father is indeed dead (*SL* 299). Only two daughters remain; St. Leon learns that Julia died shortly after her fiancé's father forbade their marriage because of a rumor that the alchemist was still alive. Like Dante's most execrable father, St. Leon's "unnatural appetite" for the benefits pursuant to alchemy causes him to "feed on the vitals of all I love" (*SL* 147), even as he deflects responsibility for his behavior onto Zampieri's gift ("the guilty cause of all this mischief" [*SL* 358]). With reference to Ugolino's gruesome eternal punishment ("it was but suitable that it should be brought home to my own bosom, that it should tear and distract my own brain!" [*SL* 358]), Godwin portrays the immortal St. Leon not as a "citizen of the world," but as an aberration of domestic and social bonds: a "repulsive power" that effectively reverses the direction of generational inheritance by consuming what has been offered by his children (*SL* 346). So freed from the "fetters" (*SL* 299) of mortality, Reginald pursues his individual life rather than submitting to the continuity of the generations. Despite his earlier protestations to the contrary, he is in fact—like Ugolino—as much a traitor against his kin as he is against the generationally figured mechanism of perfectibility.

In *St. Leon*, alchemy transforms the conjectural individual of *Political Justice* into a fictive character that demonstrates the former's incompatibility with the "great community" of species (*SL* 426). Nor are *St. Leon*'s many references to "species" incidental to the novel's critique of immortality. In fact, they speak directly to Godwin's dismantling of a central assumption of *Political Justice*: that the individual is the basis of progress. Godwin's contemporary Erasmus Darwin helps to clarify the implications of this shift from the biological necessity of old age to the articulation of "massified" identities (McLane 215). The grandfather of Charles Darwin, Erasmus was one of the leading intellectuals of eighteenth-century England. Like his famous descendant, he was a respected botanist and naturalist; and his pioneering texts on the sexual reproduction of plants, *The Botanic Garden* (1789–1791) and *Zoonomia* (1794–1797), were similarly concerned with the gradual perfectibility of species. Darwin's major works employ scientific exegesis and poetical figuration to explain how the "perpetual variation" (*Z* 1:487) of sexually reproducing plants is in fact superior to asexual modes of reproduction. For example, Darwin writes that the propagation of plants by graftings, cuttings, or runners creates a series of cloned offspring with attributes identical to the (unequivocally male) parent: "This paternal offspring of vegetables, I mean their buds and bulbs, is attended with a very curious circumstance; and that is, that they exactly resemble their parents, as is observable in grafting fruit-trees, and in propagating flower-roots" (*Z* 1:487).

In the manner of Darwin's asexually reproducing plants, Godwin's vision in *Political Justice* describes a homogeneous society of self-perpetuating, identically benevolent individuals—like so many cuttings. St. Leon himself is obviously intended as just such an ageless, asexual example of the erroneous premise of *Political Justice*: that the life of an individual is identical to that of the species. In both cases, the logic of synecdoche ensures that the individual is cloned without material difference from species. The space of difference, of speculation, and indeed of fictionality is collapsed in favor of the perfectly referential individual—an immortal, bio-allegorical facsimile of the collective. The immortal protagonist of *St. Leon* is a perfect example of Darwin's self-propagating plants: his changeless perpetuity makes him capable of creating only new, ostensibly younger, versions of himself. The coincidence of Darwin's description of asexual beings in his posthumously published long poem, *The Temple of Nature; Or, The Origin of Society* (1803) with St. Leon's situation is striking:

> Birth after birth the line unchanging runs,
> And fathers live transmitted in their sons;
> Each passing year beholds the unvarying kinds,
> The same their manners, and the same their minds.
> (*Temple*, canto II, 106–110)

This resonance is also pertinent to Godwin's famous valuation of the "domestic and private affections" in the preface (*cum mea culpa*) to *St. Leon*, which he deemed "inseparable from the nature of man . . . it is better that man should be a living being, than a stock or a stone." In this often-cited passage, Godwin's reference to a "stock" (defined in the *OED* as a "hardened stalk or stem of a plant, a rhizome"; "a stem in which a graft is inserted," in addition to "the type of what is lifeless, motionless, or void of sensation") has not yet been acknowledged as a conspicuous allusion toward mechanisms of asexual reproduction in plants and its relevance to human life-course as posited by Darwin.[21]

If the immortal St. Leon takes on an "atavistic" connotation (as Mulvey-Roberts has argued [*Gothic* 29]), it is important to note that Godwin portrays this in a specifically Darwinian sense. Moments after receiving his "grand acquisition" (*SL* 186), St. Leon remarks that "for me the laws of the universe are suspended; the eternal wheels of the universe *roll backward*; I am destined to be triumphant over fate and time!" (*SL* 188, emphasis added). Once again, Reginald misunderstands the true import of what he says: the reversion he undergoes is not that of rolling backward into youth (merely its appearance), but rather retrogression into a biologically degenerate form of being. He literally becomes "another creature" (*SL* 186), alienated from the developmental advances of his former "community of species" (*SL* 426). Like Darwin's association of solitude with asexual reproduction, the degeneration of immortality arises from the "selfish and solitary advantage" (*SL* 227) bestowed upon the alchemist. In place of the liberating escape from the fetters of sex and senescence Godwin promised in *Political Justice*, the alchemical reality of immortality effectively transforms Reginald from a sexual to an asexual organism—a being for whom succession, variation, and hence perfectibility is utterly impracticable.

Rather than a symptom of his "possessive individualism," as Mulvey-Roberts argues (*Gothic* 43), St. Leon's refusal to communicate the *elixir vitae*'s formula is, instead, a product of his *inability* to transmit this knowledge. Although St. Leon's grounds for denying the reader his alchemical secrets may be partially altruistic (such knowledge "would be detrimental to society" [*SL* 43]), the Darwinian resonances of Godwin's novel imply that his refusal is an obligatory manifestation of his unproductive perennialism. Even when it might have served his benefit (to save Marguerite from her final wasting illness, for example), St. Leon admits that he is less reluctant than powerless to share what he knows: "the elixir in question might not, *or rather could not*, be imbibed by any other than an adept" (*SL* 230, emphasis added). Like Zampieri, Reginald is now capable only of the unvarying life of paternal transmissions. The elixir thus symbolizes the obstruction of several forms of succession: biological, intellectual, and, most significantly, readerly. By withholding this crucial piece of information—how St. Leon is able to evade the onset of old age—Godwin's protagonist blocks readers' ability to entertain hypotheses about the narrative action's plausibility. Most importantly, it disrupts readers' traversal of the empathetic gap between the real and the fictional made possible by speculation. As Reginald himself exclaims, after first quaffing the elixir: "It is so different a thing to conceive a proposition theoretically, and to experience it in practice!" (*SL* 348). Godwin's protagonist comes to represent the asocial perpetual being imagined in "Of Health"—an objectification of the individualist excesses of both alchemy and the Godwinian anarchy prescribed in *Political Justice*.

Just as "Of Health" is no afterthought to *Political Justice*, neither is the final section of *St. Leon* merely appended to the closed system of the narrative. Critics have disparaged the novel's baggy "gothicity," particularly in its final volume, where tedious and "repetitious self-revilings by the hero . . . only expose the lack of coherence in the overall conception" (Kelly 235). But such repetition, I argue, actually recapitulates the novel's critique of immortality, particularly its Darwinian association of eternal life with asexual reproduction. Following several well-intentioned but doomed philanthropic ventures, St. Leon is imprisoned (for the second time) by the remarkable misanthropist Bethlem Gabor. As in the passage quoted at the outset of this chapter, he has aged considerably without his alchemical apparatus.[22] He is liberated from prison by an attacking army—led, improbably, by his son Charles, now aged thirty-two—and from his true bodily age by drinking the elixir once again. Deceived by this new companion's youthful appearance (St. Leon appears to be no more than twenty-two), Charles is happy to "act an elder brother's part" (*SL* 416). But St. Leon's guilt, enabled by his counterfeit youth, recalls Ugolino's gory punishment once again, "a secret worm gnawing at [his] vitals" (*SL* 425).

I was all a lie; I was no youth; I was no man; I was no member of the great community of my species. The past and the future were equally a burden to my thoughts. To the eye that saw me I was a youth flushed with hope, and panting for existence. In my soul I knew, and only I knew, that I was a worn-out veteran, battered with the storms of life, having tried everything and rejected everything, and discarded for ever by hope and joy. When I walked forth leaning on the arm of him who delighted to call me his younger brother, this was the consciousness that hunted my steps and blasted me with its aspect whichever way we turned (*SL* 425–426).

In the section "Of Generation" in *Zoonomia*, Darwin describes how the asexually reproducing tænia tapeworm "grows old at one extremity, while it continues to generate young ones at the other, proceeding ad infinitum, like a root of grass" (*Z* 1:489). Like Darwin's tapeworm, the immortal St. Leon is condemned to live an eternally divided life—exiled from domestic affections, doomed to an impossible double-act of age and youth. Gone is the excitement of transcendence; in its place rests the eternally static inertia of perpetuity, of mere repetition. His true pathology is shown by the obsessive, soliloquizing "I" evinced throughout the narrative—paradoxically, now signifier of the self no longer able to reflect any figure, any shadow, of personal identity. Smooth and bland with youth, he lacks even the appearance of character that is passively generated by age and the "fleshly autographics" of time (to use Eve Sedgwick's evocative phrase, viii). St. Leon is neither a father, a brother, a youth, nor a man, since the synecdochal individual has no past, future, or embodied identity of which to speak ("My appearance to a considerable degree told my story without the need of words" [411]). Thus it is significant that Godwin chose as the epigraph to *St. Leon* a phrase from William Congreve's popular play *Love for Love* (1695): the alchemical intervention forces the body itself to become a "liar of the first magnitude," perpetually effacing corporeal signifiers of old and young.

By the novel's end St. Leon is a degenerate and degenerating creature, eternally self-rejuvenating toward death, and condemned to the exile of eternal life: the perpetual offspring and asexual scion of Zampieri's paternal transmission. As we saw in Darwin's writings on sexual reproduction, the perpetual stasis of immortal life and permanent (and hence static) wealth eliminate the variation necessary to biological life—not just of the individual, as in *Political Justice*, but of species. "This, and not the dungeon of Bethlem Gabor, is the true solitude. Let no man, after me, pant for the acquisition of the philosopher's stone!" (*SL* 439). Rather than hampering life, old age and death in fact have a useful function: they command us to "live while we live" (*PJ* 1:526). Even as individual bodies may be prisoners of the biological limitation of lifespan, humanity as a whole is liberated by a newly conceived biopolitics of lifespan. In her recent survey of old age in Western philosophy and literature, Helen Small observes that "[w]hen we think about old age, our thinking rests on larger, but usually tacit assumptions about what a life is, what a person is, what a *good* life is, what social justice is, and much else besides" (2, emphasis in original). Godwin's *St. Leon* employs the fictional mode not only to illustrate a class of individuals—namely, the individual for whom old age is supplanted by radically prolonged life—but also to work through, and thus demonstrate the truth (i.e., the error) of his philosophical speculations put forward in "Of Health." In place of authorial speculation, the fictional mode relocates this task onto the reader, who is asked to pass judgement on the likelihood of the novel's speculative premises. The speculative quality of Godwin's narrative permits fiction to imagine classes of persons by simultaneously imagining and effacing the individual at the basis of the novel form. As a result, Godwin's second novel engages mindfully with the productive artifice of fiction to demonstrate the necessity of individual old age to the ongoing improvement of the life of species. For this reason, we might revise or at least supplement St. Leon's familiar designation as a "gothic" novel by acknowledging its speculative basis. In contrast to the perplexing "reality" of Radcliffe's "explained supernatural" or the fantastic romance of Maturin's *Melmoth the Wanderer*, St. Leon's fictional engagement with the matter of prolonged life in the 1790s testifies to its intellectual debts to both romance and realism.

To Small's list we should therefore add narrative fictionality as a method for generating thought about what it means to grow old. Margaret Gullette has aptly described how aging's "master narrative of decline" relies on a trope of entrance: "The plot of this one is peak, entry, and decline, with acceleration on the downslope . . . it's a universalizable plot" (*DTD* 161). But in place of the quest narrative implied by the archetypal *Bildungs*-narrative, the new biopolitical state of age has the potential to generate a new master plot. Early in the nineteenth century, literary and medicalized thinking complicated the notion of life as a singular journey by formulating age not as a series of inevitable stages but as a state that one may enter, languish in, exist in, or reverse, regardless of chronological age. Writers like Godwin were thus earnestly and thoughtfully engaged with not just the trope of entrance into old age but also escape from it. Indeed, "escape" is a key thematic and formal aspect of what I am calling the longevity narrative, which expresses the fluidity of normatively constructed categories of age. *St. Leon* is its first example, presenting as it does an extreme case of age as a conditional state rather than as a stage.

The *elixir vitae* thus signifies the potential openness of life-course, as articulated by medicalized discourses such as those of Hufeland or Godwin: despite all evidence to the contrary, life need not *necessarily* march steadily toward its dénouement in death. As the case of *St. Leon* shows, the lifespan of the individual is at once situated within and effaced by the continual reproduction of populations; by attempting to uncouple himself or herself from the perpetuity of species, the journeyer risks becoming an exile from all community. Although escaping old age is impossible for individuals, an escape of sorts is possible for populations. Godwin's novel illustrates how the mortal individual, condemned to a truncated life as one of "time's feeble children" (as Darwin phrased it in his *Temple*, canto IV l.338), is effectively immortalized in the long life of species.

Godwin's approaches to old age, longevity, and immortality are similar to those used by other speculative thinkers of his time. From the mechanistic view of human aging articulated in *Political Justice* to the organic view of life of *St. Leon*, his writings indicate a major shift in the conceptualization of human lifespan and its narrative correlates. By constructing his novel as a true fictional "history" of a speculative premise, Godwin disrupts the habit of reading lifespan as a closed arc, as one that begins, rises, declines, and then ends. Like Godwin's deviation into conjecture in *Political Justice*, the unresolved ending of *St. Leon* is not, as some critics have claimed, merely "arbitrary" (Brewer 11). Rather, the novel's final line enacts the characteristic openness of the longevity narrative. Following his son's marriage, St. Leon decides to retreat into obscurity for the remainder of his living days. The novel's final words, "Whatever may have been the result of my personal experience of human life, I can never recollect the fate of Charles and Pandora without confessing with exultation, that this busy and anxious world of ours yet contains something in its stores that is worth living for" (*SL* 449–450), reflect the disruption of the normative teleology of lifespan and the openness of the world created by fiction (the finite "result of my personal experience" versus the collective perpetuity of "[our] human life"). We are back again to Godwin's reverence for the "domestic and private affections" as the most vital element of life. Rather than a closed ending, its gerunds ("confessing," "living") and, significantly, the emphatic continuity of St. Leon's "yet" leave this novel open in a manner consistent with the speculative trajectory of Godwin's work, a literary choice consistent with Godwin's broader project to rejuvenate his readers' habits: here, the custom of reading narratives of long life in terms of narrative closure and decline.

Chapter 2

"In the condition of an aged person"

Mary Shelley and Frail Romanticism

Godwin's utopian portrait of "health and longevity" in *Political Justice* (2:519) and, subsequently, his novelistic revisitation of those hopes in *St. Leon* together constitute a case study of how massified life became linked to new valuations of age in the wake of Malthus's *Essay*. For many early-nineteenth-century writers, the linked concepts of aging, lifespan, and age identity provided an aesthetic scaffold for textual explorations of the modern subject—even as age acquired newly ambiguous, even paradoxical, meanings in the Romantic literary imagination. In truth, few keywords rival the preeminence of *youth* when defining a Romantic spirit of the age. When Isaiah Berlin writes that "Romanticism is the primitive, the untutored, it is youth, life" (20), we could point to Wordsworth's exclamation in *The Prelude*, "Bliss was it in that dawn to be alive, / But to be young was very heaven!" (book X, 1805 and book XI, 1850 editions, 520), or Percy Bysshe Shelley's exultation of perpetual freshness and replenishment in "A Defence of Poetry." Blake's dour figures of conventional law are superannuated almost without exception (see figure 1.1), and Byron's letters, poetry, and journals regularly announce his deep antipathy toward aging: "It was one of the deadliest and heaviest feelings of my life to feel that I was no longer a boy. From that moment I began to grow old in my own esteem—and in my esteem age is not estimable," to cite just one example (*Works* 445). Romanticism's celebration of youth is the linchpin of longstanding critical and historical narratives of this time. After all, dismantling the *ancien régime* demanded a new politics and poetics that cherished innocence over experience.

Even the rise of the novel, to use Ian Watt's phrase, reflects this spirit of the age. By the late eighteenth century, as Franco Moretti argues, "[y]outh, or rather the European novel's numerous versions of youth, bec[a]me for our modern culture the age which holds the 'meaning of life'" (4). Such vitally euphoric visions of youth were, and indisputably remain, key to Romanticism's critical and aesthetic brand. But this period's concurrent fascination with "pallor, fever, disease . . . indeed Death itself" (Berlin 17), so central to what scholars since Mario Praz have called "dark" Romanticism, should also intimate the possibility of a strain of Romanticism *against* youth. As I described in the introduction, Malthusian anxieties about population linked youth to an apocalyptic view of reproduction, viewing reproductive capacity less an antidote to national decline than its ominous, destructive wellspring. Such conspicuous fears of youth, or ephebiphobia (derived from the Latin *ephēbus* and Greek ἔφηβος: ἐπί "upon" + ἥβη "early manhood," "youth"), are directly at odds with what we might call the "youth model" personified especially by second-generation Romantics. If, as Tim Fulford argues (346), Malthus helped shape the rhetoric of Romanticism, then this chapter explores why matters of aging and older age—not simply youth—must be better understood as formative aspects of early nineteenth-century thought and its literary productions.

This chapter begins by charting how an anti-Malthusian backlash served as a catalyst for the idealization of youth often thought to undergird the Romantic literary imagination. Figures both within and proximate to the Godwin-Shelley circle also engaged visions of age that were not simply aesthetic exaltations of youth, thus revealing important complexities relating to the meaning of growing old—including its entanglement with visions of empire, disease, and the obsolescing of Romanticism itself. I am especially interested in how age, aging, and scenes of generational conflict help to chart competing visions of humanity that distinguish what I am calling "frail Romanticism" from more familiar subgenres (such as the Romantic youth model and dark Romanticism). To help define key elements of frail Romanticism, I focus on Mary Shelley, whose early fiction is discernibly attracted toward a Malthusian skepticism of youth's inherent virtue. I read *The Last Man* (1826) as Shelley's most compelling treatment of the disastrous potential of youth: from Perdita's pathologization of youth as a "fever" (*LM* 110) to Shelley's own admission that she wrote her novel "in the condition of an aged person" (*SLL* 146), this bold apocalypse narrative is decidedly motivated by anxieties around juvenility—even as it strives to negotiate the generational *ressentiment* that underpins Romantic idealizations of youth. In contrast to the bleak vision of later life that so disturbed many of her contemporaries, Shelley's novels often conceive of senescence as a viable, therapeutic, even consummate state of embodiment—a position not entirely idiosyncratic in the context of the Romantic age, as we shall see. For Shelley, the fictional mode is key to realizing such accord, if only because intergenerational *rapprochement* is strangely convolved with the apocalyptic conditions of lastness. If the circumstances of Mary Shelley's birth have powerfully influenced the critical approaches applied to her work, then this emphasis has also obscured an important, if perhaps less intuitive, concern: namely, the role of aging and old age in her novels and, thus far, these concepts' unacknowledged bearing upon the Romantic literary imagination.

Mary Shelley's Fictions of Aging

Of all Mary Shelley's early novels (*Frankenstein; Or, The Modern Prometheus* [1818], *Mathilda* [written 1820, published 1959], and *Valperga: Or, The Life and Adventures of Castruccio, Prince of Lucca* [1823]), *The Last Man* (1826) stands out as her most compelling engagement with older age—compelling because, like Malthus, Shelley reclaims senescence as a viable and creative state, but also because Shelley's ephebiphobia finds its enigmatic remedy in the midst of human apocalypse. The novel opens with an editor's introduction, dated 1818, describing how the book's pages were assembled from the recently-collected "frail and attenuated leaves" composed by the ancient Cumaean Sibyl in a cave near Naples (*LM* 5). The text of the novel that follows—*The Last Man*, set in the years between 2073 and 2100—is structured as the retrospective first-person account of Lionel Verney, whose father was once the favorite of the king before gambling away his fortune and familial legacy. Lionel grows up an orphaned youth and "lawless . . . savage" of Cumberland (*LM* 14) until he is serendipitously befriended by the unworldly and aristocratic idealist Adrian, whose parents are the former king and his wife, the resentful Countess of the new Republic (the monarchy has since been peacefully dissolved). Adrian's admirable character helps civilize Lionel's outlook, and eventually Lionel becomes his compatriot's partner in political affairs. After some years on the continent, Lionel returns to England to find both his country and inner circle in disarray: the ambitious and charismatic politician Raymond is agitating for greater power and ultimately marries Lionel's sister, Perdita. Meanwhile, Adrian's love for the Greek princess Evadne Zaimi goes unrequited and plunges him into a state of fever and seclusion.

Relief from this elaborate series of private dramas comes in the wake of Lionel's marriage to Adrian's sister, Idris; the Countess is appalled at this romantic rather than political match and leaves for Austria. Consequently the small circle of intimates—Lionel, Idris, Perdita, Raymond, and the convalescing Adrian—discover some tenuous peace and domestic happiness by establishing a pastoral paradise in the Windsor forest. In time, however, this happy situation goes awry. Having succeeded in his bid to become England's Lord Protector, Raymond sees his muscular plans to fortify national power fade with the commencement of his affair with Evadne, a transgression that catalyzes Perdita's deterioration and Raymond's own abdication from family and country. As Raymond commands the Greeks' war against the Turks, unsettling news of plague reaches Europe; as Lionel recalls, "I spread the whole earth out as a map before me. On no one spot of its surface could I point my finger and say, here is safety" (204). England gradually descends into chaos as a virulent plague sweeps clean every corner of the inhabited earth, until Lionel believes himself to be the world's last man.

Contemporary readings of *The Last Man* generally cite the Malthusian tropes of plague and depopulation without elaboration, focusing instead on the novel's gendered critique of empire or orientalized visions of plague. However, Malthusian skepticism of the youthful, reproductive body usefully complicates such readings. Alan Bewell, for example, hints toward this issue by observing how "plague stands apart from the categories that humans apply to it, even gender" (*Colonial Disease*, 322 n.2), while Steven Goldsmith reads Shelley's novel as a deliberate subversion of the "patriarchal formations of self, gender and language" typical to the "last man" poems that flourished in the first two decades of the nineteenth century (Goldsmith 296).[1] When Mary Poovey notes that "[s]ignificantly, all the destructive forces in this novel—the 'PLAGUE,' Necessity, and nature—are feminine," for example, we might stop to consider how the female body, particularly in older age, defies atemporally gendered associations of femininity and destruction (as did the "predictably female" Malthusian social body discussed in my introduction) (150).

While I do not mean to suggest that *The Last Man* is deliberately *about* old age, the novel is saturated with age-related imagery. Attending to age as a strategy of inquiry effectively foregrounds this novel's suspicion of the apparent timelessness of empire, nature, and the Romantic human subject. For example, having recently confirmed her ambitious husband Raymond's infidelity, Perdita writes him an anguished letter:

When the fever of my young life is spent; when placid age shall tame the vulture that devours me, friendship may come, love and hope being dead. May this be true? Can my soul, inextricably tied to this perishable frame, become lethargic and cold, even as this sensitive mechanism shall lose its youthful elasticity? Then, with lack-lustre eyes, grey hairs, and wrinkled brow, though now the words sound hollow and meaningless, then, tottering on the grave's extreme edge, I may be—your affectionate and true friend, "Perdita." (*LM* 110)

Perdita likens youth to a "fever"—a conspicuous pathologization in a novel about plague—and employs what we should now recognize as the youth-averse rhetoric of ephebiphobia. As her name ("the lost one") connotes, Perdita acknowledges the deficiencies of old age; yet in place of dread or sorrow at such losses, she asserts the productive value of her "perishable frame" over youth's carnal "elasticity." Perdita's own allusive affinity with Shakespeare's *The Winter's Tale* further indicates the restoration of the aged, older generation as a social ideal—a sentiment diametrically opposed to Godwin's denigration of aging as the ideopathological expression of political tyranny in *Political Justice*.

One could also read this passage as an instantiation of Shelley's generational engagement with her parents' respective intellectual projects. As we saw in chapter 1, Godwin's ostensibly universalizing view of the utopian, sexless, and thus immortal aging body in *Political Justice* is undoubtedly at its basis a male ("impregnable") one (*PJ* 2:519). By contrast, years earlier Shelley's mother, feminist philosopher and novelist Mary Wollstonecraft, had spoken of older age in *A Vindication of the Rights of Woman* (1792) like this: "Novels, music, poetry, and gallantry, all tend to make women the creatures of sensation . . . the exercise of the understanding, *as life advances*, is the only method pointed out by nature to calm the passions" (79, emphasis mine). By imagining reconciliation with Raymond in terms of the symbolic-cum-physiological onset of advanced life, Perdita borrows from Wollstonecraft's yearning for liberation from the body's compulsory sensibility. Perdita's lament resembles a Wollstonecraftian fantasy of the older woman liberated from the ostensibly loathsome bonds of youthful reproductivity. Thus Perdita effectively embodies what we might call a *recuperative* vision of aging and bodily decline, as it is in the diminished, "hollow" frame of tranquil age that hope exists for an authentic, intellectual sort of communion between the sexes.

In contrast to what Anne Mellor has described as Percy Shelley's "Promethean politics" ("Shelley" 70)—an ideology advanced not only in his great closet drama, but also in the authorial ethos implied by the "transitory brightness" of the mind's "fading coal" in "A Defence of Poetry"—for Perdita the stabilizing, Aristotelian frigidity of old age is required to damp the "inconstant wind" of youth.[2] Evidently, the "vulture" Perdita longs to escape is very different from that sent to devour Prometheus upon the Caucasian rocks. Mary Shelley's critique of this romantic ideology further coincides with the allegorical resonances of her novel's Malthusian epicenter. In contrast to Perdita, her estranged husband Raymond's "passions, always his masters" (*LM* 98) signal a strident desire for conquest squarely at odds with Perdita's "tottering" dotage, just as Raymond's perceptibly Hobbesian worldview stands in direct opposition to his wife's emphasis on the singular, bodily "sensitive mechanism." As Shelley writes, "[Raymond] looked on the structure of society as but a part of the machinery which supported the web on which his life was traced. The earth was spread out as an highway for him; the heavens built up as a canopy for him" (35). Raymond's imperial vision recalls Byron's enunciation of precisely such ideas in *Manfred* (1816–17), *Childe Harold's Pilgrimage* (1812–18), or "On this Day I Complete my Thirty-Sixth Year" (1824). In this latter poem, written shortly before the author's death, the speaker embraces the inevitability of mortality but only within the splendid context of battle:

> If thou regret'st thy youth, *why live?*
> The land of honourable Death
> Is here:—up to the Field, and give
> Away thy breath!
> Seek out—less often sought than found—
> A Soldier's Grave, for thee the best;
> Then look around, and choose thy Ground,
> And take thy rest. (33–41)

Here *The Last Man*'s Byronic hero embraces the faceless human "machinery" that fuels his sexualized, colonial aspirations at the basis of his elevation of youthful exuberance. Whereas Audrey A. Fisch reads Raymond's affair with Evadne as illustrative of "the flaw in the ideal union of Perdita and Raymond" (274), Shelley's ephebiphobic logic places Raymond and Perdita within the conflicting states of youth and age, respectively. We might further sense in their divorced outlooks of Perdita and Raymond a poignant inversion of the Miltonic vista that unfolds at the end of *Paradise Lost* ("the world was all about for them to choose," XII, 646): this estranged wife and husband, no longer "hand in hand," the ancient and the modern now the natural enemy of the other (Milton, 647).

Shelley's ill-fated couple stand at once together and apart as competing symbols of England in *The Last Man*. The disintegration of their marriage pits the stagnant but steady ancestral model (associated with conservative figures like Edmund Burke) against the mobile, colonial engine of modernity. Significantly, Shelley portrays Lionel—at first—in terms nearly identical to those of Raymond. Lionel describes how his "initial savagery . . . was daily instigating me to acts of tyranny, and freedom was becoming licentiousness. I stood on the brink of manhood; passions, strong as the trees of a forest, had already take root within me, and were about to shadow with their noxious overgrowth, the path of my life" (*LM* 14). Poised "on the brink of manhood," Lionel finds himself on a threshold far more precarious than the "grave's extreme edge" over which his sister Perdita peers. The initial rhetorical parallels of Lionel and Raymond are conspicuous, as is the foreshadowing of their divergent fates. Lionel's mercurial "acts of tyranny" are for Raymond a lasting chronic condition: "by some strange art [Raymond] found easy entrance to the admiration and affection of women; now caressing and now tyrannizing over them . . . but in every change a despot" (*LM* 37). The "canopy" over Raymond's "highway" far exceeds the "noxious overgrowth" overshadowing Lionel's modest "path." Ultimately, Raymond's cataclysmic failure as a husband and as England's Lord Protector implies Shelley's rebuke of that youthful, masculine, Romantic species of hero—Frankenstein, Castruccio, Napoleon and their ilk—who would utilize populations to realize bluntly individualistic desires.

In Perdita's letter as much as Burke's (whose *Reflections* celebrated the stability of the ancient in contrast to the destructive ethos of revolutionary innovation), the language of ephebiphobia and gerontophilia denotes a politically loaded shorthand for the pains of youth and the pleasures allied with older age. Like her father, William Godwin, Shelley had her literary engagement with Malthus through her linkage of the problematics of reproduction with those of age. We know that Shelley herself was reading Malthus in 1817 and, given the proximity of the *Essay* to both her loved ones and the intellectual climate of Britain more generally, it is not surprising that its concerns would figure in *The Last Man*: a narrative peopled by complex, composite characters drawn from her own fraught circle.[3] Critics including Frances Ferguson, Maureen L. McLane, Silvana Colella, and David Collings have demonstrated how nineteenth-century literature both registers and is shaped by the *Essay*'s concerns, and that a considerable percentage of popular fiction in the 1820s "is deeply affected by Malthusian preoccupations, fears and paradoxes" (Colella 22).

Then as now, critical responses to the *Essay* have tended to emphasize its apparent naturalization of the poor's miserable state. Yet the nature of these concerns is often reduced to thinly veiled caricature, for example, as in the pronouncements of Thomas Love Peacock's Mr. Fax ("a tall, thin, pale, grave-looking personage" [56]) in the novel *Melincourt* (1817): "Bachelors and spinsters I decidedly venerate. The world is overstocked with featherless bipeds. More men than corn, is a fearful pre-eminence, the sole and fruitful cause of penury, disease, and war, plague, pestilence, and famine" (59).[4] Walking the line between earnest précis and mocking embellishment, Peacock's inclusion of the age-inflected gender identities points to the entanglement of age in Malthusian portraits of reproduction. However, it is important to understand that one significant aspect of the "Malthusian" legacy is the articulation of unprecedented, biologically-figured ephebiphobia and, more generally, a new cultural and literary hermeneutic framework through which nineteenth-century challenges to the celebration of youth—manifest in outlooks ranging from skepticism to outright hostility—should be identified and interpreted.

Critics have noted that Shelley's fiction frequently critiques those predominating "Romanticisms" personified by her husband or father, yet, with only a few exceptions in the critical literature, Shelley's Malthusianism has been left to speak for itself.[5] We might begin to trace Shelley's own interest in age and aging in the elevated status generally reserved for older persons in her fiction. Consistent with the reverence for the aged shared by Burke and Malthus, Shelley's early novels often feature elderly characters as idealized figures of "unblamed old age" (*Valperga* 62). These aged outsiders are usually rendered as esteemed role models for, or foils to, youthful and perilously flawed protagonists: consider the sightless de Lacey or the old Irish magistrate in *Frankenstein*, or Mathilda's beloved servant Gaspar, or the benevolent aged hermit in *Valperga* described by Beatrice (in a conspicuous echo of Godwin's *St. Leon* and Shelley's own *Frankenstein*) as "an outcast of his species" (363). Reminiscent of Wordsworth's admiration for aged beggars and leech-gatherers, Shelley's fiction often presents elderly characters in terms of tranquil venerability and unwavering stalwartness—that is, as living symbols of individual constancy allied with the pastoral landscapes of enduring domestic (English) nature.

For Shelley, however, senescence is not limited to such idealized representation. Shelley's early novels also employ the aesthetics of aging as a symptom of grief or care in younger persons, women especially. For example, upon learning that her father actually reciprocates her incestuous desire, Mathilda observes that "the natural work of years had been transacted since the morning" and laments her new state: "youth vanished in approaching age . . . But it was not so, I was yet young, Oh! Far too young" (*Mathilda*, 174). Here the "natural," that is, heteronormative applications of affection and time are mutually corrupted. Mathilda's misdirected eros manifests as unseemly incestuous attachment, her "untimely decrepitude" the dreadful penalty of "precocious maturity" (to use T.B. Macaulay's phrase). At the end of the novella, the twenty-year-old resigns herself to the condition of an aged person: "I am grown old in grief; my steps are feeble like those of age, I have become peevish and unfit for life" (*Mathilda*, 208). Premature old age—reminiscent of the dangerously quickened rate of misfit denoted by age-*ing* in Malthus's *Essay*—is associated with traumatic longing, a desire or wish for that formerly happy state, now lost or corrupted, particularly in the social realm of familial relationships, affective or sexual bonds, or communal networks. As if to reflect the corruption and decay of the social relationships Shelley famously cherished, chronological identity finds itself out of joint with the typical stages of bodily temporal progression.

Yet Shelley's fiction also identifies the perverse, even malignant, influence of the past over the present using the symbolics of older age. In *Valperga*, for example, the quintessentially gothic crone Mandragola is alleged to have supernatural powers "greater than any queen" (377), a conspicuous prefiguration of Shelley's regal characterization of plague in *The Last Man*. Her chronological age is unknown and, apparently, fluid, as "[m]en, verging on decrepitude, remembered their childish fears of her; and they all agreed that formerly she appeared more aged and decrepid [sic] than now" (323). Rather than embodying the slow inertia of the past, Mandragola attests to the fact that what is old may also be capable of exerting undue, even catastrophic, influence over the present. As voiced in Percy Shelley's appalling catalogue of the demented George III as "an old, mad, blind, despised and dying king" in the poem "England 1819" (1), such a reading is easily aligned with the second-generation Romantics' distinctive suspicion of conservative ideological preferences for the past and its superannuated agents.

Biographical realities might have further complicated Shelley's sense of the intrinsic worth of older age. She remained deeply loyal to her father, William Godwin, even when his financial demands (most certainly exacerbated by unsuccessful attempts over two decades to refute Malthus) placed a palpable strain on her own marriage—a point to which I will return later in this chapter. Shelley once characterized Sir Timothy Shelley as a "struldbrug" (Fisch, Mellor, and Schor 6), a significant epithet given her father-in-law's lifelong refusal to financially support Mary and her son following Percy Shelley's untimely death in 1822; his fifteen-year prohibition of the posthumous publication of any of Percy's works; and his hope that, despite his advanced age, he might still outlive Mary Shelley and enjoy the satisfaction of never disbursing her inheritance. Suffice it to say, before (and for many years after) publishing *The Last Man*, Shelley was herself subject to the chokehold of an *ancien régime* openly hostile to the aspirations of youth. Both Shelley's life and fiction announce that some pasts and their superannuated agents might be worth exploding.

Shelley was hardly alone in her complex apprehension of the meaning of older age. In fact, a broader skepticism of Romanticism's proliferating youth culture might be seen to overlap with political, religious, and demographic fears of ballooning—and thus threatening—populations. In the decades leading up to the publication of Shelley's novels, political caricatures portraying Napoleon as an *enfant terrible*, for example, undoubtedly lampoon his famously diminutive stature but also the dangerous biological and ideological fecundity of France. In the decade preceding the publication of Malthus's *Essay*, France was regularly characterized by its insatiable appetites; judging from the horde of mewling brats in James Gillray's gruesome print "Un Petit Souper a la Parisienne, or A Family of Sans-Culottes Refreshing after the Fatigues of the Day" (1792), the French are portrayed as starving for sex as well as food. The dangerously reproductive habits of Catholicism were viewed a threat to England as well, as revealed by images prompted by the Catholic Emancipation movement of the late 1820s. The graphic murder of "Poor Old Mrs Constitution—Aged 141 years" depicts England as a supine *grand dame*, her bonnet askew, being strangled to death at the hands of a strapping Catholic youth (see figure 2.1). More generally, youthful desire is coarsely juxtaposed with elder murder in "Medical dispatch or Doctor Doubledose killing two birds with one stone" ("birds" and "stones" referring to female bodies and male sex organs, respectively; see figure 2.2), or in Goethe's *Faust* (1790–1829), in which the protagonist's overreaching excesses climax with the senseless butchery of Baucis and Philemon (an elderly couple in book VIII of Ovid's *Metamorphoses* who, significantly, embody the ritualized Classical ethos of hospitality).

The widespread iconography of fearsome children and elder murder ("gerontocide," to use Mike Brogden's phrase, 21) thus indicates the presence

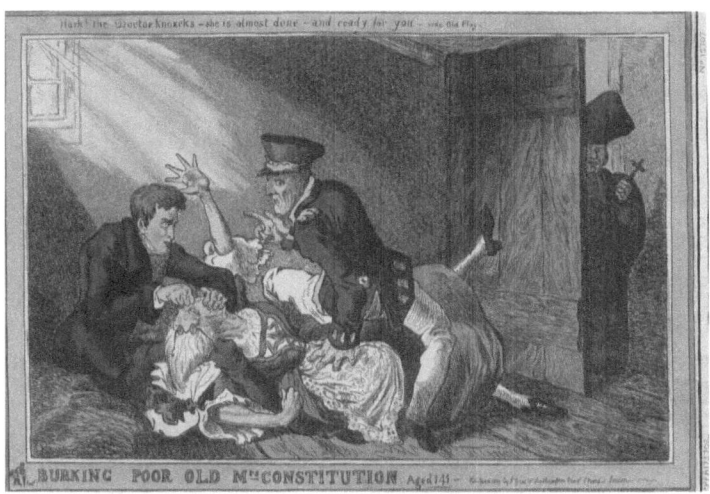

Figure 2.1. William Heath. "Burking poor old Mrs Constitution Aged 141." Published by S. Gans, London, 1829. © The Trustees of the British Museum. All rights reserved.

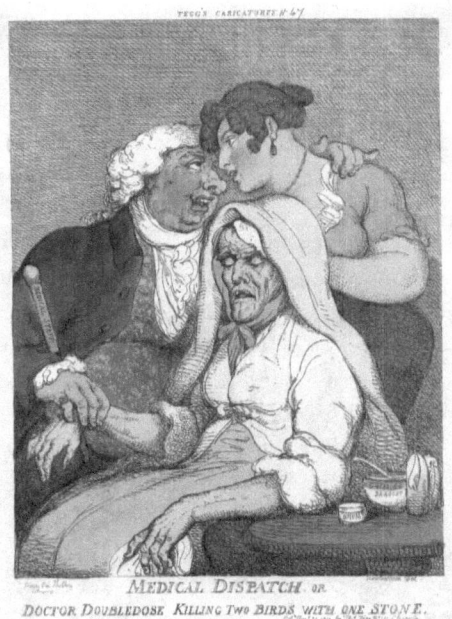

Figure 2.2. Thomas Rowlandson. "Medical dispatch or Doctor Doubledose killing two birds with one stone." Published by Thomas Tegg, London, 1810. © The Trustees of the British Museum. All rights reserved.

of a strain of Romanticism *against* youth. Yet one should be cautious of too easily "othering" these age cohorts, because for Shelley and others, youth and age could be intermingled in ways that intersected with broader, more globalized concerns of nation and empire. In the final pages of Thomas De Quincey's *Confessions of an English Opium-Eater* (1821), one nightmare stands out among the myriad pains of opium. "The causes of my horror lie deep," De Quincey shudders:

> The Malay has been a fearful enemy for months. I have been every night, through his means, transported into Asiatic scenes . . . The mere antiquity of Asiatic things, of their institutions, histories, modes of faith, &c., is so impressive, that to me the vast age of the race and name overpowers the sense of youth in the individual. A young Chinese seems to me an antediluvian man renewed. . . . It contributes much to these feelings that southern Asia is, and has been for thousands of years, the part of the earth most swarming with human life, the great *officina gentium*. Man is a weed in those regions. The vast empires also in which the enormous population of Asia has always been cast, give a further sublimity to the feelings associated with all Oriental names or images. (*Confessions* 72–73)

De Quincey's agitation, occasioned here by a keen dread of his laudanum supplier, is striking for its yoking together of Asia's "vast age" with its thronging human masses. The language and central theme of this passage of course recall Edmund Burke's definition of the sublime as that which, through pain and danger, is "productive of the strongest emotion which the mind is capable of feeling" (*Writings* 216)—as voiced, for instance, in Wordsworth's portrayal of Mount Snowdon or Percy Bysshe Shelley's "Mont Blanc." For De Quincey, the immense temporal longevity of the Orient transposes the awful sublimity of external nature onto an abstract but perceptible attribute of human beings. Whereas Shelley's "giant brood of pines" (21) around the Arve Ravine is personified by appellations of vast multitude and history ("Children of elder time" [22]), in De Quincey's *Confessions* such qualities are somehow perceptibly embodied by the "young Chinese." As his vision converges upon this instance of youth effaced and "overpower[ed]" by the inundating "antiquity of Asiatic things," the ancient, cut through as it is by race and imperial fantasy, asserts a kind of catastrophic grandeur. In this passage De Quincey glimpses an "antediluvian man renewed," a strange amalgam of senescent juvenility in which the alpha and omega of human life, the cradle and the grave of nations, share a strained coexistence. Here "youth" is effectively a living relic of an ancient national past, a palimpsest of the innumerable bodies forged and rendered over countless generations in Asia's great *officina gentium* ("workshop of persons").

Instead of dooming life, the deep time of the Orient is associated with stable and even robust sexual reproduction, in keeping with earlier assessments by Adam Smith and Jean-Baptiste Du Halde discussed in my introduction. But, as Montesquieu doubted then, such success is not all it may seem. We read that in its "vast age" Asia is "swarming with human life," a teeming *hoi polloi* rife with a peopleish pestilence endemic to its ancient stock and nature. Throughout the passage, the language of immensity ("impressive," "thousands of years," "vast empires," "enormous population") bespeaks not simply the sublimity of this thriving primeval culture—not to mention De Quincey's anxious orientalist fears and fantasies—but also the potential monstrosity of human life itself. "Small herbs have grace: great weeds do grow apace" (*Richard III* 2.4.13): the virulent "weed" that so disturbs De Quincey is the ancient race revivified in the young reproductive body of the Malay before him. The "further sublimity" of the Orient seems a consequence of this malignant generation, its vast empires relentlessly populated by a swarm of reanimated Methuselahs.

In one sense, the Malay is maligned as "a fearful enemy" for furnishing the English opium eater's laudanum dreams. But De Quincey's wrangling of population and age points toward an additional framework of meaning in this passage. After Malthus, unchecked human growth was urgently recast as a fearsome probability. Suddenly the Orient loomed large as a case of such imminent catastrophe, and Europe's own increasing numbers seemed less a boon than a liability. From the pleasures to the pains of population: the trajectory of the opium eater describes also the shifting meaning of population growth after Malthus as the antediluvian dream of complementary human and external natures found itself overpowered by the nightmare of too much youth, too many people. From rebellious Catholic multitudes to the malignant hordes of Asia, after Malthus the sublime empire of youth generated tremendous anxieties about the fate of individual and massified lives both within England and beyond its borders.

"That fatal child, the terror of the earth"

Shelley's fictional exploration of the ethical possibilities of older age has particularly suggestive potential for literary criticism and, moreover, why senescence, as a constitutive category of difference, is deserving of greater consideration in the context of nineteenth-century literature and culture. Like the passage from De Quincey above, Shelley's doubt concerning the unalloyed good of youth is evident in her treatment of age and aging within a transformed context of population. Although *Frankenstein* is often read as an allegory of unseemly creation, Victor's attachment to alchemy also cautions against unwarranted preservation. As one professor marvels, "these fancies which you have so greedily imbibed are a thousand years old and as musty as they are ancient" (*F* 31); Krempe's outrage is directed as much toward Victor's reluctance to look to the scientific innovations of the present as toward his student's incongruous enthusiasm for the "sad trash" of "exploded systems" (*F* 31). Given the centrality of alchemy to William Godwin's anarchist aspirations and, more generally, to the revolutionary élan of late eighteenth-century England, such passages imply Shelley's own skepticism of obsolete ideas that might be given new, yet treacherous, life.

Throughout the Romantic period, alchemical images continued to be wielded with exactly this kind of insubordinate enthusiasm. Percy Shelley's "Alastor: Or, the Spirit of Solitude" (1816) condenses into four lines the Romantic youth model of rebellion with the botanical vernacular of sexual procreation and literary genius:

> Oh, for Medea's wondrous alchemy,
> Which wheresoe'er it fell made the earth gleam
> With bright flowers, and the wintry boughs exhale
> From vernal blooms fresh fragrance! (672–675)

Not surprisingly, "Alastor" points toward a passage in the *Reflections* in which Edmund Burke decries those who would reject the past "as a heap of old exploded errors" (243) using a figure of alchemically induced geronticide. Burke's own fears are palpable: "By this wise prejudice we are taught to look with horror on those children of their country who are prompt rashly to hack that aged parent in pieces and put him into the kettle of magicians, in hopes that by their poisonous weeds and wild incantations they may regenerate the paternal constitution and renovate their father's life" (244). Significantly, *The Last Man* also gestures to both of these sources, but with a quiet, unambiguous relinquishment of the ardor of "Alastor": "[Adrian] seemed born anew, and virtue, more potent than Medean alchemy, endued him with health and strength" (*LM* 237). As the earlier example of Perdita indicates, Mary Shelley's emphasis on the stabilizing remedy of virtue is at variance with the compulsory innovation intrinsic to the sexualized Promethean politics of futurity.

Speaking of *Frankenstein*, McLane argues that "[t]he contest between Victor and monster, at first an agonistic doubling of individuals, becomes in this second experiment a world-historical contest between imagined populations—the 'whole human race' versus 'a race of devils' . . . He [Victor] cannot imagine his creatures *not* reproducing" (103). Thus Mary Shelley's portrayal of "The Modern Prometheus" offers a Malthusian critique and amplification of similar themes raised by Percy Shelley's *Prometheus Unbound*. In the latter text the Titan Jupiter asserts, with mistaken delight, how he has "Hurl[ed] up insurrection, which might make / Our antique empire insecure" (*Prometheus*, 3.1.8–9). However, unlike Jupiter's dismissal of his lingering ephebiphobic apprehensions—"Even now have I begotten a strange wonder / That fatal child, the terror of the earth" (19)—Victor foresees with terrible clarity the disaster imminent to the reproductive victory of his dreaded successor. As Victor nears completion of the female creature he experiences a kind of Malthusian epiphany ("the wickedness of my promise burst upon me" [Shelley *F* 145]), and his laboratory takes on the appalling outline of an *officina gentium* in which he can only imagine "the children of his creatures . . . as 'mass' and not 'individual instance'" (McLane 104). Both Frankenstein's Creature and Shelley's novel assiduously ensure the wreckage of futurity: children are either effaced or dispatched, and both aging and generational succession appear all but prohibited.

Whereas De Quincey's fears of the proliferating multitude are cast toward the Asiatic races of the Orient, Victor views premature national aging as a considerably more local concern. Although Victor's request that the Creatures remove to South America already acknowledges the impossibility of permanent exile from Europe (McLane 105), Fred V. Randel has shown that *Frankenstein* is even more immediately engaged with British geopolitical concerns regarding Ireland. Between 1760 and 1840, an exploding Irish population strained its tenuous union with Britain. "Quite literally," writes Ina Ferris, "the margins of the nation begin to press on the centre, assuming a frightening gigantism, and the population–fact begins to exceed its strictly economic dimensions" (33). Such monstrous pressure was apparent to contemporary historians as well, as expressed in Sir Richard Musgrave's two-volume *Memoirs of the Different Rebellions in Ireland, From the Arrival of the English: Also, A Particular Detail of That Which Broke Out the 23d of May, 1798; with the History of the Conspiracy Which Preceded It* (1801). This widely read, unsympathetic account of the 1798 Irish rebellion consistently links the proliferative Roman Catholic population to the destruction of social order: "it is to be feared, that they would explode, if they were more numerous, and should a foreign invasion, or any publick disturbance that endangered the State, offer them an incitement to do so. Like the winds confined in the cave of Eolus, if the pressure of the mountain was removed, they would hurl destruction" (xv). Musgrave recounts the reality of large Irish families, their teeming homes, and worrisome dietary dependency on the potato, by sounding a Burkean alarm concerning the violent uprising of a "popish multitude" (38). Such critical and historical perspectives intersect at their profound anxieties concerning the violent male's capacity for growth, an unease signaled by the age-related nomenclature attached to rebel groups as "The White Boys" or "The Right Boys."[6]

In *Frankenstein*, when Victor is overcome by the Creature's potential reproductive future, it is because he understands how, like Malthus's matron, he might be accused of a "most atrocious selfishness" (*F* 149). To produce a potentially "malignant" race would be like creating another Ireland, a population whose rampant growth was perceived as gravely injurious to the well-being of England ("Had I a right, for my own benefit, to inflict this curse upon everlasting generations?" [*F* 144]). Given the geopolitical valences of fearsome youth and reproduction at Shelley's time of writing, it is no accident that Victor unwittingly drifts toward Irish shores following his drowning of the female creature's "relics" (*F* 149). The country's populous and agitated masses are promptly reconstructed. Victor is soon bombarded by the local inhabitants: "several people crowded toward the spot"; "[Victor] perceived the crowd rapidly increase;" "a murmuring sound arose from the crowd as they followed and surrounded me" (*F* 151). Nevertheless, Victor's surprisingly civil treatment by the local inhabitants (this despite reasonable suspicion that he is Henry Clerval's murderer) appears to point out only the barbarity of Victor's botched attempts at reproduction, not that of the Irish crowd. Speaking of this encounter, Randel notes that *Frankenstein* "temporarily posits, then decisively discredits, the stereotypes about the Irish that supported England's colonial dominance" (484). If Shelley refuses such national typecasting, however, she continues to rely on the characterizing force of imagined populations. Accelerated growth—for both the individual and the crowd—retains its potential as a threatening and readily othering sign.

We can thus read *The Last Man* as a continuation of the ephebiphobia first explored in *Frankenstein*. As the catastrophic effects of a global plague begin to take hold, *The Last Man* imagines not just nations but also a world beset by too much youth. This nightmare of maturity reaches its climax during Raymond's war against Asia, specifically in Evadne's death scene. Like Perdita, Raymond's jilted mistress is a strange hybrid of youth and age. But unlike Perdita (who wishes to emulate the non-reproductive virtues of the aged), Evadne embodies the destructive accelerations of the dangerously aging nation. Her "consuming fire" and "crimson . . . fever"—at once signifiers of both plague and youth—are inseparable from the Promethean-cum-Malthusian disaster she summons against her former lover (142). "This is the end of love!—Yet not the end! . . . the instruments of war, fire, the plague are my servitors! . . . Fire, and war, and plague, unite for thy destruction—O my Raymond, there is no safety for thee!" (142). As if to gesture to her sources, Evadne effectively paraphrases the *Essay*'s massifying catalogue of the apocalyptic "vices of mankind" pursuant to excess youth. As Malthus writes:

> The vices of mankind are active and able ministers of depopulation. They are the precursors in the great army of destruction; and often finish the dreadful work themselves. But should they fail in this war of extermination, sickly seasons, epidemics, pestilence, and plague, advance in terrific array, and sweep off their thousands and ten thousands. Should success be still incomplete, gigantic inevitable famine stalks in the rear, and with one mighty blow levels the population with the food of the world. (Malthus 56)

In both texts, the active destruction signaled by the reproductive body is matched only by the sublime methods of extermination that youth in too-great numbers can summon out of external nature itself. Indeed, Shelley's novel utilizes plague precisely for its Malthusian connotations of the consequences of human growth. Significantly, *The Last Man* adopts Malthus's language above immediately following Lionel's recognition of the global reach of plague ("ere this men have gone out in sport, and slain their thousands and tens of thousands" [205]), as both authors evoke the sublime culling described in Revelation 5:11 ("and the number of them was ten thousand times ten thousand, and thousands of thousands"). Evadne's transformation into a dangerous masculine combatant further recalls Malthus's fear of the gentleman-warrior for whom the privileges bestowed by gender and youth make the soldier a conduit of an apocalyptic human sublime. Raymond's mistress presents a doubled vision of the generative capacity of youth and the catastrophic grandeur of the ancient; in her defection from Greece to Turkey, Evadne embodies the transitioning ages of the sluggish West and its revivified geographical other. Hence Lionel's meditation on Evadne's prematurely expressed old age, deeply reminiscent of the language of Perdita's letter ("the lost, dying Evadne" [*LM* 142], "her eyes . . . sunk deep" [143], the compounded hollowness of "hopeless love and vacant hopes" [142]). Only thirty, "her limbs had lost the roundness of youth and womanhood," an observation further aestheticized by his adaptation of Shakespeare's Sonnet 63: "Crushed and o'erworn, / The hours had drained her blood, and filled her brow / with lines and wrinkles" (143).

Physiological youth thus provides the basis by which the Promethean "empire of . . . passion" (*LM* 78) is made manifest on a massified scale. Shelley deploys plague deliberately for its Malthusian connotations of the consequences of human growth. However, in spite of Perdita's and Raymond's respective species of misery, *The Last Man* asserts that community is nevertheless possible—even in the face of, or indeed, because of, the catastrophic outcomes of youth. If plague destroys, it can also animate. Shelley portrays the beneficiaries of these circumstances as an unruly fleet of Americans, those "relics of that populous continent" who suddenly return to Britain by way of Ireland seeking a new site for survival (231). It is as if De Quincey's Asiatic scenes have returned home, "seizing upon the superabundant food" and methodically exhausting the natural resources of each spot they settle (231). The reanimated populations of Ireland and North America are now imperially mobile and ready to swarm the decrepit ship of England Lionel famously describes in the novel's first paragraph. As war breaks out with the Irish-American invaders, Shelley's inverted narrative of colonial exploitation demonstrates the futility of the language of empire once the imperial, linear narrative of history collapses. In the face of plague, the new world becomes a "relic" of the old world, which becomes the new world, and so on. In an interesting reversal of Malthus's observation that "we shall not be surprised that the fears of the timid nations of the South represented the North as a region absolutely swarming with human beings" (86), Lionel's wary admission that there "was room enough indeed" (232) for this unanticipated influx of "relics" to his newly youthful homeland inscribes Malthus's observation onto the peri-apocalyptic England of *The Last Man*. Just as Victor fears in *Frankenstein*, a noxious bloom of youth returns to Europe with boundless malignancy.

In contrast to Raymond's idealization of war described earlier, Adrian is disgusted by its reliance upon generations of human grist. "I have learnt . . . that one man, more or less, is of small import, while human bodies remain to fill up the thinned ranks of the soldiery; and that the identity of an individual may be overlooked, so that the muster roll contain its full numbers" (124). In this battle, however, it is unclear as to which side tarries with the burden of national aging. Indeed, in its proclivity for war it is Raymond's Western empire resembles the gathering swarms more traditionally associated with the East. Adrian's objection points out the discomfiting reciprocal relationship between de- and re-population: so long as human bodies remain, the antisocial success of population ensures a perpetual war of generation(s).

Writing the Universal Calamity

It might be tempting, at this point, to label Shelley's politics of aging as "conservative," aligned as it is with skepticism of Romanticism's Promethean aesthetics. However, in spite of superficial similarities, Shelley's fourth novel deviates from the ephebiphobic commitments of *Frankenstein* by decoupling the linkages between decline and decrepitude, youth and novelty. Where Malthus can only imagine the catastrophe pursuant to youth, *The Last Man* ultimately retreats from biological fatalism by exploring how the physiological virtues of older age might be grafted onto youth as a socializing principle. Yet what hopefulness exists for overcoming youth's dangerous potential? Although the word "hope" is mentioned more than 245 times throughout the novel—almost twice the frequency of the term "plague" (130)—the text reaches contradictory conclusions. Does the reader allot greater significance to the assertion that "Hope is dead!" (244), that it is a "precious freight" (214), or that "we were not born to enjoy, but to submit, and to hope" (312)? In the final pages of the novel the fable of Pandora's box, in which the "inspirited loveliness" of a "young Hope" gives way to "decrepitude" and death, strongly suggests not only the pessimism of Shelley's examination of social relations in the context of population, but also of *The Last Man* itself (245).

The novel's latter half exploits an important and unremarked Malthusian irony: just as plague is the "medicinal vial" Lionel seeks to restore England's health (185), so does senescence promise a means of survival amidst the catastrophe of youth. This paradox is at the root of exclamations concerning the apparent universality of aging in the face of plague. "The world had grown old, and all its inmates partook of the decrepitude. Why talk of infancy, manhood, and old age? We all stood equal sharers of the last throes of time-worn nature . . . there was no difference in us; the name of parent and child had lost their meaning" (252). Despite the indisputable dejection of such a passage, phrases like "[w]e all stood equal sharers," "there was no difference in us," convey an emergent—if subdued—sense of community fostered by the assumed perspective of older age.

The Last Man is Shelley's most personal novel, so it is not surprising that such impulses might germinate in moments of biography. Critical discussions of *The Last Man* inevitably refer to a journal entry dated May 14th, 1824, as a turning point both in Shelley's profound grief following the death of her husband and in the composition of her *roman à clef*. On that day she writes, "The last man! Yes I may well describe that solitary being's feelings, feeling myself as the last relic of a beloved race, my companions, extinct before me . . . And thus has the accumulating sorrows of days & weeks been forced to find a voice" (*SLL* 146). Less familiar is an intriguing entry made the next day following that morning's news of Byron's death in Missolonghi:

> A new race is springing about me—At the age of twenty six I am in the condition of an aged person—all my old friends are gone—I have no wish to form new—I cling to the few remaining—but they slide away & my heart fails when I think by how few ties I hold to the world—Albe, dearest Albe [Shelley's nickname for Byron], was knit by long associations—Each day I repeat with bitterer feelings "Life is the desert and the solitude—how populous the grave." (146)

Feeling acutely isolated and longing for the "populous" land of the dead (less a Malthusian slip than a citation of her mother Mary Wollstonecraft's favorite, Edward Young's long poem "Night Thoughts" [1743–5] and the epigraph to Godwin's *Essay on Sepulchres* [1809]), Shelley makes an arresting assertion of her own accelerated senescence. This rarely cited lament is generally overlooked in pursuit of more overtly apocalyptic visions figured in *The Last Man*, but Shelley's language of alienation is significant to a novel concerned with the possibility of sociality in the face of total catastrophe. To link lastness with old age would have been roughly consistent with her historical moment, since throughout the eighteenth century "to live long meant, most often, loneliness among a generation of strangers" (McManners 73), an attitude Byron's own Childe Harold knew well:

> What is the worst of woes that wait on age?
> What stamps the wrinkle deeper on the brow?
> To view each loved one blotted from life's page,
> And be alone on earth, as I am now. (canto II, XCVIII)

Two years after her disheartened entry, Shelley's despair evolves into muted hope for the socially renovating capacity of senescence. Toward the novel's end, Lionel recounts how a false prophet "exultingly proclaimed the exemption of his own congregation from *the universal calamity*" (*LM* 318, emphasis mine)—a phrase used here to refer to the fictional plague, but also one, significantly, that also appears in Jonathan Swift's *Gulliver's Travels* to describe the interminably aging Struldbrugs. I find it striking that for Swift and Shelley alike, the "universal calamity" forces a state of age-worn sameness upon a population, be it Swift's tiny class of fantastic miserable beings or the global populace of *The Last Man*. By altering the calamitous terms of this condition, Shelley portrays human suffering not as a product of protracted old age but, rather, of the state of individual youth. In the course of writing this novel, Shelley develops a striking double vision of her own: if youth and age can inhabit the self-same being, then perhaps it is possible for generations to coexist in the sphere of social relations.

The Last Man therefore demonstrates a biographically consistent commitment to the referentiality of fiction as a means of overcoming generational *ressentiment*. A poignant example is evinced in Merrival, the "little old astronomer" (172), which Morton D. Paley and Anne McWhir (in her introduction to the Broadview edition of Shelley's novel) have separately identified as Shelley's most critical portrait of Godwin. I mention Merrival here because, importantly, he also signifies the proximity of Malthusian ideas to *The Last Man*. To the extent that William Godwin is his referent, Merrival is less a sketch of the esteemed author of *Political Justice* than the pitiful shadow "Poor Godwin" had become by the early 1820s (James 376). As described in my introduction and chapter 1, Malthus had struck a very public blow to Godwin's radical idealism, effectively arresting the latter's career as a public intellectual. While he continued to write novels and children's books, Godwin would never again occupy his former celebrity status. Twenty-two years after Malthus first published the *Essay* (and four popular editions later), Godwin's long-awaited response finally materialized. His six-hundred-page *Of Population* is an embarrassing blot: a witless, blistering *ad hominem* attack antithetical to the collegiality of the 1801 *Spital Sermon*, wherein Godwin had once praised the clarity of Malthus's argument. An anonymous review in the *Edinburgh Review* (1821) strikes close to the bone: "The present work [Godwin's *Of Population*] proves, either that we were wrong in our estimate of [Godwin's] powers, or that they are now greatly impaired by time. It appears to us, we confess, to be the poorest and most old-womanish performance that has fallen from the pen of any writer of name, since we first commenced our critical career" ("Godwin on Malthus" 362–363). The reviewer—almost certainly Malthus himself—persists by further diminishing the now stroke-afflicted Godwin as "an old scold" with "enfeebled judgement" (363), the author of "work which we had thrown aside" (364). Nor was this the only review written in this tone. *Of Population* was unanimously viewed as woefully late, ineffectual, and saturated with an obsolete Jacobin spirit entirely alien to the day.

This sad final act of the Godwin-Malthus debate illustrates how Shelley's father was conspicuously out of time in the years immediately preceding the composition of *The Last Man*. It is likely, then, that Godwin's radical idealism inspires Merrival's unseemly optimism that the disastrous plague will make way for an earthly paradise "in an hundred thousand years" (*LM* 172):

> [Merrival] came now to announce to us the completion of his Essay on the Pericyclical Motions of the Earth's Axis, and the precession of the equinoctial points. If an old Roman of the period of the Republic had returned to life, and talked of the impeding election of some laurel-crowned consul, or of the last battle with Mithridates, his ideas would not have been more alien to the times, than the conversation of Merrival. . . . [He] talked of the state of mankind six thousand years hence. He might with equal interest to us, have added a commentary, to describe the unknown and unimaginable lineaments of the creatures, who would then occupy the vacated dwelling of mankind. We had not the heart to undeceive the poor old man; and at the moment I came in, he was reading parts of his book to Idris, asking what answer could be given to this or that position. (227)

The facetious tone in which Lionel compares Merrival's "announce[ment]" to the immateriality of archaic politics or speculative evolution evinces how, in both age and ideology, Merrival is profoundly "alien to the times." But unlike Ryland's contemptuous rebukes ("And we shall of course enjoy the benefit of the change" [*LM* 172]), Lionel strives to see through this temporal detachment to imagine something like a shared moment of simultaneity.

Lionel's wife, Idris, meets Merrival over the astronomer's book-in-progress, dwelling at once in the midst of and apart from the catastrophic inevitability of plague: an act that patches together a moment of communion within the destructively productive futural logic of species generation ("six thousand years hence"). Shelley does not rescue either Godwin or Merrival from their exile. Yet *The Last Man*, a conspicuously belated contribution to its own subgenre of apocalypse narratives, demonstrates a form of transgenerational sympathy—evident in Shelley's creation of a fictional narrative motivated by a perception of parity with her aged father that endeavors to anatomize their mutual suffering. This momentary convergence of old and young illustrates both a literal and figurative instance of growing older together, facilitated in the social (if fictional) spaces generated by reading and writing.

Nevertheless, Merrival's demise also testifies to the fragility of such simultaneity. Confronted with the death of his wife and children from plague, Merrival "felt the system of universal nature which he had so long studied and adored, slide from under him, and he stood among the dead, and lifted his voice in curses" (239). Like unaccommodated Lear upon the tempestuous moor, Merrival's ultimate trauma is the recognition of his own futility: "The breeze scattered the grey locks on his temples, the rain drenched his uncovered head, he sat hiding his face in his withered hands . . . age, grief, and inclement weather, all united to hush his sorrows. . . . He died embracing the sod" (239–240). Merrival, Godwin, Shelley herself: *The Last Man* imagines each as the tormented relic of a beloved race. By fictionally inhabiting Merrival's suffering, Shelley partially recuperates Godwin even as her *roman à clef* chides his presbyopic fixation on the far-off future.

This string of critical concerns—lastness, loneliness, and the productive imaginary of aging and senescence—reminds me of Karen Chase's description of why older age presents such a compelling opportunity for literary analysis. Bodily aging "encourages an irreducibly private subjectivity to confront its own last days. Part of the ethics of our scholarship is indeed to overcome the gap of loneliness" (Chase, "Coming" 38). Likewise for Shelley, for whom seeing oneself "in the condition of an aged person" obscures the definitional properties of chronological age in the pursuit of a complex, often agonizing sympathy among age classes. It is no coincidence, then, that older age figures as a therapeutic balm throughout this particular fictional exercise—a kind of ethical strategy, perhaps, that distinguishes Shelley's Romanticism in *The Last Man* from the youthening Promethean model in which she nevertheless remained enmeshed. If Evadne is an emblem of the dangers of accelerated aging, then the recuperative potential of older age becomes the means by which community can be cultivated in the midst of the Malthusian crisis. For these reasons, we can conclude, numerous characters of miscegenated youth and age populate *The Last Man*: from the elderly Martha, who aids her ailing community by bringing food to the ill in the midst of the plague, to the Countess (Lionel's formerly contemptuous mother-in-law), who becomes a valuable political advisor as the crisis worsens, these aged "archons" link social—indeed, immunological—stability with a remarkable egalitarian sensibility (213). *The Last Man*'s fictional aperture generates a compound space for growing older together, assuaging the generational *ressentiment* of the Promethean youth model.

In the midst of gathering reports of "physical evils" (177), Lionel employs the riddle of the Sphinx to contemplate the nature of ancestral progression, individual aging, and massified perpetuity. Watching his son play amidst a small group at the grounds of Eton, he muses:

> Here were the future governors of England; the men, who, when our ardour was cold, and our project completed or destroyed for ever, when, our drama acted, we doffed the garb of the hour, and assumed the uniform of age, or of more equalizing death; here were the beings who were to carry on the vast machine of society . . . It was not long since I was like one of these beardless aspirants; when my boy shall have obtained the place I now hold, I shall have tottered into a grey-headed, wrinkled old man. Strange system! riddle of the Sphinx, most awe-striking! that thus man remains, while we the individuals pass away. Such is, to borrow the words of an eloquent and philosophical writer, "the mode of existence decreed to a permanent body composed of transitory parts; wherein, by the disposition of a stupendous wisdom, moulding together the great mysterious incorporation of the human race, the whole, at one time, is never old, or middle aged, or young, but in a condition of interchangeable constancy, moves on through the varied tenour of perpetual decay, fall, renovation, and progression." (*LM* 179–180)

Lionel's retrospectively narrated passage effects a strange sort of *hic jacet* for those doomed youth who will never "assum[e] the uniform of age"; "[h]ere were," of course, reads for Lionel as "here lies" given his backward-looking recounting of events. He marvels at this "strange system" of generational succession by citing the riddle of the Sphinx: an ancient Greek mythological creature who asked Theban travelers—Oedipus most famously—"What creature has four legs in the morning, two in the afternoon, and three in the evening?" The answer, of course, is a man, whose lifetime of crawling infancy, upright youth, and debilitated old age are collapsed into the duration of a single day. The real "puzzle" of the Sphinx relies upon the strangeness of man's instability of identity: over the course of a life, implausibly related creatures nevertheless inhabit the self-same being (Lionel identifies himself both with the "beardless aspirants" before him and the "grey-headed old man" he will become). In its rejection of radically fractured states of age— either their antagonism, as per Malthus, Percy Shelley, or Blake, or their incongruity, as per De Quincey or Burke—the Sphinx becomes a figure of Shelley's resistance to the Romantic youth model in its imagination of the lived simultaneity of multiple states of age.

This citation of Burke's ancestral framework—the tragic "drama" of the individual is effaced by the maintaining hand of "renovation, and progression"—does seem calculatedly old-fashioned. Lee Sterrenberg has argued that Lionel's ventriloquization of Burke is decidedly "ironic" (332) and, certainly at this point in his story, Lionel is not yet fully cognizant of the calamitous manner in which the human drama will be rent from the "stupendous wisdom" of external nature. Lionel envisions the boys as "future governors," but the ill-fated machinations of Raymond resonate in his belief that they will "carry on the vast machine of society" in this all-too-neat mechanical "replacement" model of successive generation. This passage presages the shipwreck of hopes for human progress put forward in Volume I, a disaster later literalized by the sinking of the enormous Irish-American gunship heralding the violent return of the colonies to their British homeland. The fate of "th[at] huge unwieldy machine," whose capsizing demonstrates the grim human ends of "the true spirit of reckless enterprise," is proof against Burke's outdated certainty of generational succession (232). In place of comforting ideas of society's interchangeable constancy, the great *officina gentium* is destined to produce a monstrous surplus of individuals ("transitory parts") that cannot all be placed at Nature's inhospitable table. Rather, the inevitable excess incurred by the perpetuation of the permanent body of species threatens the very possibility of growing old together.

As Oedipus discovers, the essential clue necessary to unraveling this skein is one's apprehension of the interconnectivity between generations (a knowledge Oedipus will, of course, eventually perceive he has unintentionally yet fatefully exploited). Against the riven biopolitics of war, Shelley's novel ultimately negotiates these contrasting temporal models of collective subjectivity by exploring the possibility of integrating temporalized classes in a social vision of miscegenated youth and age. Shelley thus posesses a double vision of her own: if youth and age can inhabit the self-same being, then perhaps it is possible for generations to coexist in the sphere of social relations. This strangely hopeful ideal reaches its culmination in Adrian, an idealized rendering of Shelley's husband, Percy. Adrian's character is drawn in almost wholly contrasting strokes to those of Raymond: he never marries, remains childless, and spends his youth civilizing Lionel's "savage" tendencies. In the face of the Irish and American invaders, Adrian mobilizes his troops' compassion rather than their fury with emphatic reminders of the intrinsic humanity of "these misguided men" (235). Against enormous odds, in this moment of colonial reversal Adrian flattens generational geographies to appeal to the simultaneity of a universal humanity: "Shall man be the enemy of man, while plague, the foe to all, even now is above us, triumphing in our butchery, more cruel than her own?" (236). He is, for a time, successful in linking old and new worlds where Perdita and Raymond once fell apart—"The two forces mingling, unarmed and hand in hand"—until the plague impartially diminishes both sides to dust (236).

Adrian is, in essence, something close to an ideal Malthusian subject: a young person—male at that—who strives to behave according to the physiological virtues of the old. Like Martha, his mother the Countess, and even the doomed Perdita, following his recovery from a mysterious (and in this novel, unavoidably symbolic) fever, Adrian is revived to embody the non-reproductive merits of the older woman. For the remainder of the novel, Adrian abrogates the simple pathologization of either youth or age by behaving in terms of the physiological simultaneity of age metaphorized in the Theban Sphinx's riddle. Unlike his former *amour* Evadne, Adrian is salvaged from an injurious destiny by rejecting the reproductive impulses of his youth. Responding to Ryland's terror upon realizing the inescapable virulence of the epidemic ("great God, who talks of help! All the world has the plague!" [191]), Adrian provides a succinct and poignant example of this ironic sort of hope in the face of decline. His gentle, smiling response—"Then to avoid it, we must quit the world" (191), or even Lionel's earlier plea, "Let us leave 'life,' that we may live" (171)—conveys the Malthusian horizon of the novel's Godwinian aspirations. In spite of the inevitability of growing old, *The Last Man* implies that humanity can rest assured of nature's inescapable regeneration—even if, as Shelley's Malthusianism intimates, it is at the expense of the very human agent that makes hope possible.

Mary Shelley's early fiction, and especially *The Last Man*, demonstrates its Malthusianism not only by reserving a privileged place for older age but also in Shelley's self-positioning at the center of this fictional encounter. Malthus's *Essay* determines how a population could at once be young but also dangerously aging, thus complicating the hegemony of the individual subject that has come to represent the familiar Romantic lyrical "I." In step with this attention to population, Malthusian thought makes clear the need to make room for old age; for Shelley, it is only in the fictional domain that the promise of sociality intrinsic to senescence can be realized. In keeping with the logic of the Sphinx's riddle, perhaps we might read the architecture of Shelley's novel as reflective of its commitment to realizing the simultaneity of past, present, and future. The "Introduction" is dated 1818 and the speaker (a Shelleyan figure whose referentiality to the author—or even gender—is famously indecipherable) describes the discovery of the Cumean Sibyl's cave. Like the Sphinx, the Sibyl is herself a mythological figure being implicated in the matters of age and longevity; after asking for as many years of life as she could hold grains of sand, she spurns Apollo's advances—she is granted her wish for long life but suffers, like Tithonus, without accompanying youth. Shelley was no doubt attracted to such a figure, not simply as a conceit for an otherwise improbable narrative (a tactic typical to the last man subgenre), but for the Sibyl's composition of prophecies "in the condition of an aged person." The speaker of Shelley's Introduction is thus tasked with the translation of "the frail and attenuated Leaves of the Sibyl" to generate in the present the story of the future foreseen in the ancient past (*LM* 5). As Barbara Johnson has noted (265), the narrative begins by assembling the elements of the future perfect mode by fashioning the present into a mutual destiny to come or, as Paul Ricoeur puts it, the "present [that] will have been the beginning of a history that will one day be told" (1:260). Such a move immediately entangles the temporality of the reader in the process of novel-reading, elaborating further the shared world of the *roman à clef* in which the stuff of fiction is coextensive with that of "real" life: that is, where life is always aging toward decay.

As in Burke's *Reflections* and Perdita's letter, Lionel too records his account for an imagined young reader. "And who will read them? Beware, tender offspring of the re-born world—beware, fair being, with human heart, yet untamed by care, and human brow, yet unploughed by time—beware, lest the cheerful current of thy blood be checked, thy golden locks turn grey, thy sweet dimpling smiles be changed to fixed, harsh wrinkles!" (*LM* 341);

"If I were to dissect each incident, every small fragment of a second would contain an harrowing tale, whose minutest word would curdle the blood in thy young veins" (*LM* 312). Lionel preserves the "radical hope" (to use Jonathan Lear's phrase) that his memoirs will be one day encountered by sympathetic future generations. Simultaneously, Shelley's reader encounters *The Last Man* both as a relic of the past and, now more than ever, a herald of the precarious future.

Shelley's complicated sense of hope is nowhere more evident than the novel's final pages. Now that a year's waiting has not brought him a single instance of the human company he longs for, a gray-haired Lionel meditates on his loneliness and desire to leave Rome. "My person," he exclaims, "with its human powers and features, seem to me a monstrous excrescence of nature" (365): a statement reflective of the superfluity of one accretion—human life—to the function and future of nature (not to mention an almost exact repetition of St. Leon's laments I described in chapter 1). Though it presents, no doubt, a definitely gloomy sort of hope, Lionel realizes that his fate will remain unchanged if he does not leave. In response to the sublime animation of the ruins around him Lionel sets off to "find what I seek—a companion" or, failing this, to carry on "anchoring in another and another bay" (366). Though he claims that "[n]either hope nor joy are [his] pilots," Lionel betrays a nascent desire whose significance at this late stage of the novel cannot be overlooked, if only because its familiarity is unmistakable (367). "I long to grapple with danger, to be excited by fear, to have some task . . . for each day's fulfilment" (367). Even the face of inescapable ruin, at the limit point of all aesthetic possibilities of decay, the last man on earth exhumes the youthful seeds of motivation by which his species was once wrecked. Shelley's fourth novel concludes with this embryonic hope that the ruins of humanity, in all its generative potential, might secure the chance to suffer its downfall again.

Frail Romanticism

This chapter has shown how the biopolitics of youth and age, evident in the wide scope of literary, political, and economic texts concerned with the relationship between generations, shaped prevalent strains of Romantic culture. In its difficult capitulation to the inevitability of decay, *The Last Man* stands out as an exemplar of what I call "frail Romanticism": a muted tendency evident within the broader Romantic imagination that concedes the vulnerability of the body and the corporeal limitations of the human subject. Distinct from the Promethean youth model (which tracks closely, albeit imperfectly, with the euphoric investments of conventional Romantic thought) and the literary subgenre of dark Romanticism (which reflects prevailing fascinations with the supernatural, irrational, demonic, and grotesque, as G.R. Thompson and others have described),[7] frail Romanticism is defined by a high consciousness of the temporalized infirmity of the flesh: not, however, for the purposes of summoning the gratuitous cruelties of Nature nor censuring the delusive ambitions of fallen man. Instead, frail Romanticism is defined by its commitment to imaginatively, even tenderly, concretizing the divergent temporalities of individual selfhood and the strangely inconceivable facts of bodily aging, lateness, and lastness. In adopting the term "frailty," I do not undercut the robust tenets of Romanticism as a cultural and aesthetic movement, nor should use of this term insinuate some measure of judgment as to how productively a text instantiates its Romantic tendencies. Rather, frail Romanticism calls attention to the diversity of literary explorations of senescence and its aesthetics at this time: not only for the ways such infirmities constitute their fictional referents, but also the ways such thematics provide insight into the transformative declensions of a larger literary movement.

The Last Man is, in several senses, a narrative written in the position of an aged person: be it Lionel, Shelley, or Shelley's own inhabitation of the characters (drawn from "real" referents or otherwise) reanimated in the pages of her fourth novel. Yet frail Romanticism abounds elsewhere too: in the tenuous physicality of Keats's body and body of work, be it Apollo's "d[ying] into life" (line 130) in the abortive generational drama of *Hyperion* (1818–20); or the senescent fixations of Walter Savage Landor's long career ("On His Seventy-Fifth Birthday" [1853], "Memory" [1863], and the living elegy "To Wordsworth" [1834]).[8] Multiple entries in Charles Lamb's vital *Essays of Elia* (1823) and *Last Essays of Elia* (1833), such as "The Convalescent," "A Complaint of the Decay of Beggars in the Metropolis," "The Superannuated Man" and others, engage the thematics of frail Romanticism I have described. Furthermore, reading them in this vein highlights the precursor role of frail Romanticism with respect to the emergence of the mid-century cult of the invalid, and the genre of illness writing motivated by what disability studies scholars might call the "crip" sensibilities of figures like Harriet Martineau, especially her *Life in the Sickroom: Essays by an Invalid* (1844).[9] Dorothy Wordsworth's *Grasmere Journals* (1800–2) are crowded with attention to aged figures throughout; of her brother William's work there is more to say in the next chapter. Indeed Wordsworth himself—his body as much as his career, which underwent an eclipse much like William Godwin's—was as much a marker of frail Romanticism as was his notorious attention to figures of older age throughout his career ("Simon Lee," "Resolution and Independence," "The Old Cumberland Beggar," "Animal Tranquility and Decay," or the late "Sonnet to an Octogenarian," to name a few). In 1839, De Quincey published a series of biographical essays in *Tait's Edinburgh Magazine*, exposing (and at times, no doubt, embellishing) the human foibles of his former mentor, where he confessed he "learned gradually that [Wordsworth] was not only liable to human error, but that, in some points, and those of large extent, he was frailer and more infirm than most of his fellow-men . . . I viewed him now as a mixed creature, made up of special infirmity and special strength" ("Sketches" 636). In this excerpt and throughout the curious essay from which it is drawn, De Quincey struggles to apprehend multiple frailties: of his once-admired role model, and the literary movement Wordsworth himself so infamously outlived.

As the examples I have outlined show, there exists enough variance among formulations of generational relationships—as contrary states, contradiction, opposition, and so on—that the common critical and pedagogical shorthand for this period demands re-evaluation. This is especially true given the sheer numbers of nineteenth-century literary writers who are themselves, in several senses, miscegenated figures of youth and age. The complicated Romantic afterlives of figures like De Quincey, Sara Coleridge, John Clare, Thomas Carlyle, Charles Darwin, Anthony Trollope, and George Eliot—to say nothing of Wordsworth's notorious 1850 revision of his earlier Romantic idealism—should be proof enough that this period cannot be sensitively reduced to an infallible empire of youth. Indeed, the fraught aesthetics of youth, aging, and senescence reveal the range of inventive analyses critics might bring to reading the early-nineteenth-century politics of age and generation. One thread we might follow is the Romantic invention of aging as a modern social crisis.

Chapter 3

George Eliot's Aging Bodies

> Cold Pastoral!
> When old age shall this generation waste,
> Thou shalt remain, in midst of other woe
> Than ours, a friend to man . . .
>
> —John Keats, "Ode on a Grecian Urn"

Could Keats have dreamed that his study of the Grecian urn might be repurposed by rather more familiar successors, a breed of historian for whom the strange "foster-child" (line 2) under consideration was not merely a quiet object, or an insensible sylvan scene—but the "[f]or ever panting" (27) life of Romanticism itself? By mid-century, the Romantic vision was indisputably out of breath. Mary Shelley's *The Last Man* had prophesied that youth would devastate the promise of her generation; yet old age would visit the Romantics twice over. First came Wordsworth's wasting after his golden decade following the publication of *Lyrical Ballads* (1798), which earned Percy Shelley's condemnation of the "double ghost" in "Peter Bell the Third" (1819, published 1839): "who has lost / His wits, or sold them, none knows which . . . / And though as thin as Fraud almost— / Ever grows more grim and rich" (157–161). The second strike was an apparent reversal of the very aesthetic delineations of Romanticism itself (or, as poet Robert Browning called it, "a set of miserable little expedients, just as if they represented great principles"), combined with Wordsworth's revivification into a most eminent Victorian (Browning, "Essay" 578).[1] "Ode on a Grecian Urn" ends on a note as prophetic as it is elegiac. By 1850—the year of the elder poet laureate's death at age eighty—Romanticism was itself in desolate shape: a parched epoch whose youthful aspirations left it burned to the socket.

The immortal urn Keats imagines stands apart from the bodily finitude of its viewer, foiling the corporeal erosions of human time with the paradoxically ancient scenes of the "for ever young" (27). Old age, writes Keats, can only "waste" this generation of ekphrastic beholders: but in what sense, exactly, is old age so incommensurate with youth? Here "waste" conveys the inevitability of physical ruination while conjuring images of unseemly consumption and useless employ. If we read Keats's reference to "generation" as an allusion to his own Romantic cohort, perhaps the urn itself also stands forward as a tribute to—or remnant of—such wasted Romanticism, looking ahead to bodily senescence and to a dramatically transformed cultural aesthetic. In contrast to the Romantic youth model discussed in chapter 2, Victorian self-fashioning was regularly accomplished under the standard of older age. One need only compare the feathered lines and blooming tones of Keats's portraits with the venerable beard that overwhelms Charles Darwin's iconic *cartes de visite* to judge how the discursive iconography of age differently inflects these two nineteenth-century periods. Experience bests innocence, maturity preempts juvenility: with few exceptions, by the time of Wordsworth's death, the validity of the Romantic youth model had been all but rescinded.

Literary historians have generally accepted this vision of cohort replacement, in which the Victorian succession of Romanticism reflects the progression of adolescence by older age.[2] Certainly this idea holds true to some extent. Karen Chase associates the Victorian period with the inception of "the elderly subject" (*Victorians* 6), a discursive category effected by the emergence of gerontology as a field of medical study, as well as literature, painting, and journalism that was increasingly prompted by shifting demographics and new cultural aesthetics of old age. Linking this fulsome embrace of an aged identity to the very public aging of Queen Victoria, who ascended the throne in 1837 at age eighteen and ruled until her death in 1901, Chase argues that Victoria's bodily age and the Age that bears her name—its seriousness, earnestness, and espousal of its monarch's widowhood—"reflects a public that was also aging and, for the first time, in numbers and influence great enough to constitute a dominant perspective" (159). While retropolated demographic data illustrate that a significant change in British society's age structure was not apparent until approximately 1890 (as discussed in my introduction), the Victorian perspective was—and to large extent remains—synonymous with older age, as if the ancient face of Keats's urn was no longer the font of extreme alterity but rather "a friend" to a more sympathetically elderly beholder (Keats, 48).

Yet this chapter challenges that familiar generational account of nineteenth-century literary history by demonstrating the Victorians' profound interest in the complex linkages of youth and age, specifically through the evocative idea of "waste." As both a literal and figurative phenomenon, waste has generated considerable scholarly discussion of late, so let me be clear as to my focus here. For one, waste has been associated with the toxic alterity of filth (as William A. Cohen and Ryan Johnson have described, for example, in Zola's naturalistic aesthetics of filth in the city).[3] The expression of agedness as a form of diseased or disgusting excess is, unfortunately, not unheard of at this time: the dementing Mrs. Affery in Dickens's *Little Dorrit* is belittled as nothing more than "a heap of confusion" and a "piece of distraction" (733), while Trollope's narrator in *The Fixed Period* (1882) describes the elderly as "a scum of the population,—the dirty, frothy, meaningless foam at the top" (129).[4] Alternatively, notions of aging as a form of *economical* waste are also present in a range of texts, from Godwin's portrait of economical and physiological hoarding in *St. Leon* to more recent models of age-related change described in terms of "gain" and "drain" (Baltes and Smith 124). Oscar Wilde's *The Picture of Dorian Gray* also features here, but is remarkable for the way Lord Henry Wotton flips the logic of aging as expenditure on its head. Whereas Shakespeare's sonneteer bemoans lusty expenditures as "[t]h'expense of spirit in a waste of shame" (Sonnet 129, 1), Lord Henry questions the stockpiling of virtue if its only purpose is to lengthen life into the "hideous puppet[ry]" of older age (Wilde 187). "Don't squander the gold of your days," he implores Dorian; "I thought how tragic it would be if you were wasted. For there is such a little time that your youth will last—such a little time" (187). In Wilde's novel, waste is figured as the unjustifiable safeguarding of youth against the luscious imperatives of consumption, a physio-economic binary materialized, of course, in Dorian's severance of his gorgeous life from the telltale portrait banished to the attic.

Given my book's interest in the aesthetics of embodiment that shaped nineteenth-century visions of aging, my focus here is, instead, on waste as a *physiological* principle: that is, an inevitable, dissipative force derived from the mid-century discovery of the second law of thermodynamics (i.e., the process of entropy). Catherine Gallagher has shown how the cross-cutting of physiology by economics was one of the lasting innovations of the Malthusian paradigm shift for the way it identified "the interconnections among human life, its sustenance, and modes of production and exchange" (*BE* 35). It is this somatic, physiological connotation of waste and its relevance to nineteenth-century thinking about aging that this chapter attends to. George Henry Lewes's widely read *The Physiology of Common Life* (1859–60), for instance, describes physiological change throughout the life-course as a ongoing dialectic between "Waste" and its counterpart "Repair." His long discussion of age and aging in chapter XIII ("Life and Death") imagines life as a dynamic equilibrium of physiological forces in which youth and age are *mutually* susceptible to the physiological processes of waste and repair. In place of antagonism or opposition, Lewes's vision of waste and repair makes the individual body a lifelong composite of youth and its antithetical, often abject, Other. Here gain and loss (and their associated metaphors of production, conservation, and expenditure) constitute a facet of the Malthusian array of bioeconomical concerns Gallagher describes. To live is to participate in one's ongoing ruination, a hypothesis that underpins Lewes's discussion.

Although recent studies by Chase, Kay Heath, Claudia Nelson, and Teresa Mangum have demonstrated the value of reading Victorian novels through the lens of age studies, Lewes's contribution to the Victorian imagination of aging has not yet received sustained consideration. Recent works by Suzanne Raitt and Anne-Julia Zwierlein have begun to explore the ways in which reanimated interests in vitalist concerns (such as Hufeland's, described in chapter 1) provided a framework for accelerating concerns regarding premature aging, especially toward the century's end. Yet my interest in Lewes's underdiscussed work is piqued by the ways in which his vision of "waste" speaks not only to increasingly medicalized visions of aging at this time, but also to the extensive interdisciplinary network of ideas that inform novelist George Eliot's portrayal of older age and the aging body.

This chapter revisits the now-familiar intellectual bonds that join Lewes's scientific investigations with Eliot's literary writing by focusing not on the novelist's well-known uptake of Lewesian psychology but on the physiological principles that formed the basis of her domestic partner's influential treatise.[5] Published shortly after Lewes's *The Physiology of Common Life*, Eliot's novel *Silas Marner: The Weaver of Raveloe* (1861) conveys a multifaceted concern with economic and bodily wasting. Reading *Silas Marner* through the Lewesian lens of waste and repair, I argue, offers a new entry point into our understanding of the concomitance of growth and decay in Eliot's novels more generally: not only in terms of their representation of the body's temporal fate, but also in how the Victorian novel might be said to imagine how we might live alongside the indelible fact of aging.

The first part of this chapter explores Lewes's understanding of aging and the life-course as an ongoing dialectic of youth and age, one characterized by their *mutual* susceptibility to the forces of waste and repair—a stark contrast to the individualized ages of life model, and one that makes use of an explicitly terrestrialized lexicon that takes the long life of the earth as an unexpected but vital cognate for aging human beings. In the second part, I demonstrate how Eliot adopts and adapts waste and repair as a means of portraying the shared states of old and young throughout *Silas Marner*: as a physiological principle that elucidates the strange reality of Silas's "withered and shrunken" life (129), and then reinvented as a social ethic that dramatizes the sharing of resources between old and young. Where *The Physiology of Common Life* considers the concurrence of youth and age in the individual, however, Eliot transmutes this simultaneity into the social milieu of intergenerationality. In *Silas Marner* and elsewhere, this living synthesis of old and young finds its concrete figuration in the image of the interlinked hand: a somatic locus that reads both as a fleshly *cipher* of the reciprocity of youth and older age, as well as the tactile *means* through which such intergenerational contact might be realized. While this imagery underscores Eliot's ethical, allegorical, and probably moral agenda in *Silas Marner*, the final part of this chapter posits how waste and repair offers a new entry point into our understanding of the concomitance of growth and decay at this time: not only as it concerns the Victorian conceptualization of human aging, but also the literary-historical imagination of the aging nineteenth century itself.

Lewes and the Physiology of Aging

The mid-century discovery of the second law of thermodynamics had direct implications for physiological conceptions of the human body. If, as the second law maintains, transformations of energy incur an inevitable loss of heat even as total amount of force in the universe is conserved, then the body must be subject to a similar dissipative principle. As Suzanne Raitt explains, "The apocalyptic fears unleashed by the 'new physics' played themselves out in texts which used the body as an image for the universe, and death was imagined simultaneously as an inevitable biological process that was the result of a gradual accumulation of waste (unusable energy), and also as an event which could be carefully negotiated by the management of waste substances and of the internal economies of the body" (1).[6] Since death marks the conclusive failure of repair to recompense the expenditures of waste, thrift and efficiency (as much civic as biological principles in Victorian social thought, as Tim Armstrong notes [43]) came to constitute the ideological foundations of the Victorian "economy of the body" (Pick 6).

The modest scholarship that exists on this topic invariably refers to Herbert Spencer as the exemplar of this Victorian thermodynamic hypothesis of life. "Repair is everywhere and always making up for waste," Spencer writes in *Principles of Biology* (published in 1864), and elsewhere he speaks of the "waste Universe" (*Autobiography* 470)—a lexicon "still current" in 1922 and cited enthusiastically by Freud (Small and Tate 127). Yet earlier sources exist and, most importantly for my purposes, possess a compelling proximity to the Victorian novel. Five years prior to Spencer's discussion in *The Principles of Biology*, Lewes had already directed extensive consideration toward the principles of waste and repair in the human system. Published in two volumes between 1859 and 1860, *The Physiology of Common Life* imagines life as a dynamic equilibrium of physiological forces: "In every living organism there is an incessant and reciprocal activity of *waste* and *repair*. The living fabric, in the very actions which constitute its life, is momently yielding up its particles to destruction . . . unless the substance of your body, which is wasting, be from time to time furnished with fresh food, Life flickers, and at length becomes extinct" (1:4–5; emphasis in original).[7] Waste and repair constitute the two reciprocal nodes underlying the fate of what Lewes calls "the living fabric" (1:7), an aptly material and, by this point in the industrializing nineteenth century, strongly commodified image of the body, a conceptual history that invokes both Thomas Carlyle's 1836 *Sartor Resartus* (and its Professor of "Things in General," Diogenes Teufelsdröckh) as well as Andreas Vesalius's 1543 anatomical treatise *De Humani Corporis Fabrica* (*On the Structure of the Human Body*).

Significantly, especially in light of Eliot's *Silas Marner*, Lewes immediately personifies the principle of bodily repair as an assiduous weaver, whose exertions serve to restore monetary and bodily coffers alike. "Hunger sits at the loom, which with stealthy power is weaving the wondrous fabrics of cotton and silk . . . the money we all labour to gain is nothing but food" (1:2). On one hand, Lewes warns against a life dominated by the refusal to repair: by forgoing the virtues of temperance and efficiency, the *bon vivant* accelerates the bodily fabric's decay. But Lewes's formulation also implies how excessive thrift—the monkish self-abnegation that would withhold one's means of repair—effects identical symptoms. "The man who takes no food, lives, like a spendthrift, on his capital, and cannot survive his capital. He is observed to get thin, pale, and feeble, because he is spending without replenishing his coffers; he is gradually *impoverishing* himself, because Life is waste. . . . We cannot say how long such a spendthrift life may continue" (1:8–9).⁸ Whereas early Romantics often took modern economic life as anathema to bodily preservation and authentic selfhood (consider Wordsworth's "Getting and spending, we lay waste our powers" in "The World is Too Much With Us," (line 2; 1802, published 1807), by contrast, the Victorians' tidy bookkeeping accepted intake *and* output, rather than the steady incursion of energy from nature, as the means of sustaining life's weft and warp.

Life is waste: this striking refrain throughout *The Physiology of Common Life* underpins Lewes's hypotheses concerning human aging in chapter XIII ("Life and Death"). Rather than ignoring aging or apprehending it as the mere antagonist to growth, Lewes reads physiological change over time as a symptom of the shifting equilibrium of expenditure and restoration. "If the Repair were always identical with the Waste, never varying in the slightest degree, Life would be only terminated by some accident, never by old age. But the Repair is never thus nicely balanced with the Waste" (2:369). Remarkably, in place of the organicist model of progressive development (what I.A. Richards once described in a visual rhyme as the equivalence of "knowledge and growledge" [Abrams 169]), Lewes views the individual body in terms of a lifelong composite of growth and decay.⁹ A distinctive suite of metaphors reflects this view. "Manhood," he writes, is "a sort of table-land in life, but its limits are very variable . . . The balance of waste and repair is tolerably even" (2:365). In speaking of a tableland, appeals to its literal connotations—a broad, elevated, level expanse of ground such as a plateau—but probably also to its figurative meaning, that is, as "an elevated or level state or position" (*OED*, "tableland"). (Such evocative language is also used, for example, by George Eliot to describe the whiggish Mr. Bult in *Daniel Deronda* [1876], who is observed to possess "the general solidity and suffusive pinkness of a healthy Briton on the central table-land of life" [200].) While such terrestrial visions of aging persist in our own time (we might speak of being "over the hill," or of older age as the "decline" or "downslope" of life),¹⁰ Lewes's insistence on variability complicates longstanding striations of childhood, youth, manhood, and old age: "Every organism has its limits of duration which are definite and inevitable; we cannot assign these limits with precision, any more than we can assign the precise stature which an animal will attain; we can only fix boundary-marks within which the duration is possible" (Lewes 2:364).

Lewes's model diverges considerably from the conceptual scaffold of the pyramidal "stages" of life (or *Lebenstreppe*, a widespread visual representation of human aging in Europe and North America since the seventeenth century; see figure I.1). For Lewes, "Old Age" occurs when "[t]he balance [of waste and repair] begins to lean; the movement of Assimilation slackens, and Death slowly advances. The limits of this epoch are the most variable of all" (2:366). It is the shifting preponderance of waste and repair, not the passage of chronological time as such, that really determines the fleshly phenomenology of human aging. Lewes's insistence on the heterogeneity of older age (rather than the universalizing chronology of age categories), and the relationship between waste and repair it indicates, requires a language of aging that is capable of encompassing this synchronicity. As he writes, "we must remember that Time is only *our* conventional means of measurement; and that the phenomena measured are in no sense regulated by Time" (2:365).

To my ear, tablelands, limits, boundaries, and epochs do not immediately call to mind geriatrics so much as a kind of corporeal landscape or topography.[11] It is as if *The Physiology of Common Life* is deliberately evoking analogical ideas in Charles Lyell's *Principles of Geology*, a text first published in 1830 and one with which Lewes was intimately familiar. Thirty years earlier Lyell had demonstrated that longer-term forces like erosion and sedimentation had brought about changes in the earth's composition (as opposed to the cataclysmic disasters separated by periods of stability, as Georges Cuvier's earlier catastrophist paradigm had held). Lyell's language of natural history, which told the story of a dynamically and radically ancient Earth, should sound familiar: "the renovating as well as the destroying causes are unceasingly at work, the *repair of land being as constant as its decay*" (1:473; emphasis added). Speaking specifically of earthquakes in his concluding remarks to volume 1, Lyell writes:

> [I]t appears . . . that the constant repair of the dry land . . . [is] secured by the elevating and depressing power of earthquakes. This cause, so often the source of death and terror to the inhabitants of the globe . . . and fills the earth with monuments of ruin and disorder, is, nevertheless, a conservative principle in the highest degree, and, above all others, essential to the stability of the system. (1:479)

Lyell's understanding of the ongoing reciprocity of geological renovation ("the constant repair of the dry land") and waste ("the earthquake that produces monuments of ruin and disorder") sees a tolerably even balance of these forces over time—an ongoing reciprocity of forces that together make up what we now call the "deep time" of the earth.[12]

It is therefore intriguing to note how the central physiological principle in *The Physiology of Common Life* effectively builds on Lyell's geological sense of erosion, building, and gradual change. (The *OED* also indicates that "stages," a key word in age studies and for representations of aging, acquired geological implications following Darwin.)[13] By asserting that "*Life is the dynamical condition of the Organism*" (2:356, emphasis in original), evidently a direct analogical chain exists between physiological and geological visions of time. What purpose is served by these geological remnants? Noah Heringman has described how the landscapes of literary Romanticism regularly drew on geological metaphors and the "material textuality" of rock itself in order to "clearly confron[t] the coexistence of economic and aesthetic imperatives in a social context" (12). Consider the example of Wordsworth's ancient leech-gatherer in "Resolution and Independence," who incorporates both the ossification of "extreme old age" and the senescing personification of the cragged landscape in which he is situated:

> As a huge stone is sometimes seen to lie
> Couched on the bald top of an eminence; . . .
> Such seemed this Man, not all alive nor dead,
> Nor all asleep—in his extreme old age . . . (57–58, 64–65)

Wordsworth's youthful speaker names the profound alterity both of old age and the inorganic matter it resembles ("a huge stone . . . Such seemed this Man") by readily transmuting the leech-gatherer's aged body "into a geological lexicon" (Heringman 37). In fact, the tendency to view older age as "not all alive nor dead" is anything but an eccentric nineteenth-century archaism. Hospital culture in our own time regularly invokes similar figurations of age-hardening; consider the pejorative label "rock" applied to chronically ill, bed-ridden patients, while "the rock garden"—frequently used with reference to traumatic brain injury or geriatric care wards—indicates the speaker's sense of those patients' utter inertness.[14] In such cases, the aged body is viewed in terms of the absolute subjugation of organic life by inanimate stoniness, a disturbing twenty-first-century reiteration of what Heringman calls the "trauma of solidification" (103).

Yet "Resolution and Independence" and, to a much greater extent, *The Physiology of Common Life* ultimately reject this dismal, single-faceted understanding of aging. In fact, Lewes's geological framework underscores his interest in the profound interconnectedness of inorganic and organic realms, particularly in the context of age-related change. Lewes directly references geology in chapter XIII as a means of better understanding the "familiar mysteries" of human aging:

> Men who are thrilled at the tokens of the past life of man, when they see, or read of, buried cities, Palmyra, Nineveh, or Yucatan, tremble with no delicious awe at the tokens of the past life of this earth, when they stand in a quarry, or ramble through a geological museum. Yet surely the crystal is not less mysterious than the plant; the ebb and flow of the tides not less solemn than the beating of the human heart? (2:354)

Lewes weighs familiar organicist metaphors—the plant, the heart—against the promise of rocks and tidal amplitudes as means of describing life, to conclude that we are more akin to the crystal than we care to admit. In place of the vital principle, *The Physiology of Common Life* looks to the continuities of geology to account for the heterogeneity of aging and older age. Consequently, Lewes circumvents the moralizing imperatives of early and mid-century physicians like Christoph Hufeland or Jean-Pierre Flourens, protogeriatricians who saw lifespan as a fixed (if plausibly extended) parabolic arc unless exhausted by hygienic blunders like excessive food and drink or opium consumption. Borrowing from Barnard Van Oven's memorable formulation in *On the Decline of Life in Health and Disease* (1853), Lewes states, "Man begins in a *gelatinous*, and terminates in an *osseous* condition" (2:368, emphasis in original). If the ossifying, aging body remains an artifact of time's passing, it is a relic that confounds the simple distinction between organic and inorganic forms.[15] Nor is Lewes entirely idiosyncratic in this regard. Such vital intermingling of inorganic and organic life forms occurs in Charles Darwin's early consideration of coral atolls, ecological systems that he proposed were produced by the immensely slow process of land subsidence and the accumulation of living polyps upon the calcareous matter of the dead—like Wordsworth's leech-gatherer, who grows out of and on top of the stony landscape in which he lives. Reading Lewes's words today, we might also note how nineteenth-century networks of exploitation have led to profound dramatizations of failed resource sharing across time and generations: failures that take the form of devastated coral reefs and, indeed, the geopolitical horrors that preceded the 2015 destruction of Palmyra. Not all things can repair or evolve.

I mention these examples to briefly contextualize Lewes's description of human aging among a constellation of other disciplinary discourses—literary, geological, ecological—that likewise posited the coexistence of ostensibly incommensurate states of life. The reality of common life depends on the dynamic simultaneity of apparently oppositional systems, be they biology and geology, organic and inorganic life, life and death. Lewes adopts this approach precisely because it grants a means by which to account for the otherwise confounding simultaneity of physiological growth and decline over time. Lewes's evocative opening to chapter XIII, whose allusive description of a recently deceased human body quotes Wordsworth's "Sonnet Composed upon Westminster Bridge, September 3, 1802," corroborates this overarching textual strategy. "The man whom we loved and honoured, who an hour ago was full of energy, affection, hope, and endeavour, is now lying an inert mass before us, insensible, inanimate. . . . *All that mighty heart is lying still*" (2:345, emphasis added). The personifying impulse of Wordsworth's sonnet ("Ships, towers, domes, theatres and temples lie / Open unto the fields, and to the sky" [lines 6–7]; "The very houses seem asleep" [13])—renders London a vital organ of England (indeed, if population is any consideration, the city pinpoints the industrializing world's "mighty heart" as well) that is itself anthropomorphised again, as Lewes's conceit indicates, as a being in repose. This key instance of intertextuality recapitulates the pattern we have seen thus far and indicates, as the next part of this chapter will elaborate, how thoroughly Wordsworth is interwoven throughout Lewes's and Eliot's respective treatments of aging.

By this point, Lewes's relationship to classical nineteenth-century organicism bears conspicuous signs of strain. In her indispensable study *Darwin's Plots*, Gillian Beer describes how nineteenth-century evolutionary thought shares with organicism its central maxim of "irreversible growth and succession" (Beer 106). Yet neither paradigm satisfactorily accounts for the existence of old age and its complication of the growth plot; old age generally signals existence beyond reproductive life, and aging beyond reproductive capacity is not easily mapped onto species development. Indeed, older age manifests an uncomfortable problematic of growth by extending development beyond the "fully adult" subject that Beer takes as the "default" Victorian subject (107). While Beer observes that "[e]volutionary assumptions of irreversible change have reinforced our observation of individual growth," she adds, "it is salutary to remind ourselves that the two concepts are not inevitably connected" (104). For example, Beer names "recrudescence" (101) or reanimation as one phenomenon that defies the assimilative impulse of cumulative growth—significantly, a topic addressed by Lewes in chapter XIII, and a phenomenon that usefully describes Silas Marner's strange revival in the second half of Eliot's novel. Writes Lewes, "[t]he microscopic animals known as Rotifers become, to all appearance, dead, when the water of the moss in which they live is evaporated; and in this state of suspended animation they may remain for years, recovering their energy on the addition of a little water. . . . [T]hey are not dead in these cases, and they do not decompose" (2:346).

The composite life of the rotifer—like the leech-gatherer, not all alive nor quite dead—is thus an extreme example of the dynamic simultaneity of waste and repair, and indicates organicism's crucial inability to account for both the existence of old age and how senescence undermines the dominant Darwinian growth plot associated with the Victorian period.[16] All this has immediate consequences for our understanding of nineteenth-century aging. Lewes's writings develop the interdisciplinary account of how the Victorians were shaped not only by a multifaceted view of old age, but through their attempts to come to terms with living with aging itself. In fact, waste and repair provide a cogent conceptual framework that helps explain just why older age at this time appeared, as Karen Chase recently put it, "frequently unpredictable and as often unstable . . . a transient rather than a permanent condition" (*Victorians* 4).[17] Because the fluid reciprocity of waste and repair defies irreversibly forward-looking trajectories, the literary imagination is especially well positioned to explore such counternarratives of the human life-course. Consider representations of premature or accelerated aging in the literature of this time in which the body appears at odds with chronological age, as it does for aged children like Jenny Wren in Charles Dickens's *Our Mutual Friend* (1864–65), or Thomas Hardy's Little Father Time in *Jude the Obscure* (1895). Or the inevitably disastrous attempt to divorce youth from older age, as in Dorian's body-portrait division in Oscar Wilde's *The Picture of Dorian Gray* (1891), or in Anthony Trollope's bizarre novel *The Fixed Period* (1882), which depicts the consequences of state-sanctioned euthanasia at 67-and-one-half years of age. Or even in the restoration of the riven lives of disparate generations in the context of the collective social body, an impulse evident in a number of Eliot's novels (particularly the Burkean metaphor of *mortmain*, "the dead hand"). Insofar as nineteenth-century literature may be said to grapple with the increasingly common reality of living with aging, waste and repair indicate the ways in which old and young, like past and present, do exist—and perhaps must exist—as contiguous rather than oppositional modalities. Lewes's discussion of aging in *The Physiology of Common Life* therefore constitutes a vital envoy between science, medicine, and the public realm, to say nothing of his lasting and intellectually generative domestic partnership with perhaps the foremost novelist of this period.

Waste and Repair: The Weaver of Raveloe

In spite of a growing number of studies on Victorian old age and midlife, few discussions of aging in Eliot's work exist. Those that do address aging tend to fixate on Dorothea and Casaubon's May-December marriage in *Middlemarch* (as if age disparity, "a fine bit of antithesis," as the painter Naumann observes, was the *raison d'être* of marital misery [*MM* 172]).[18] Such readings, while usefully descriptive, indicate the need for more historically sensitive, interdisciplinary critique of what appears to be the inescapably didactic symbolism of older age. Gallagher's demonstration of the centrality of Malthusian thought to Victorian discussions of organic life offers a cogent bridge between physiological and literary engagements with the meaningful representation of aging at this time. Eliot figures prominently in *The Body Economic*, and Gallagher convincingly demonstrates the Malthusianism of concerns with childbirth and overpopulation in Eliot's early short fiction (*Scenes of Clerical Life*, 1857–8) and her last novel, *Daniel Deronda* (1876). And yet, as the introduction and first two chapters of this book have established, one essential facet of Malthus's legacy involves the matter of human aging—a convergence of topics that, Lisa Niles's discussion of Gaskell's *Cranford* (1851, 1853) notwithstanding, has largely escaped notice. As my discussion of Lewes and Lyell indicates, the sharing of resources across time and the dramatization of generational resource rights as a form of waste and repair, are a further dramatization of a Malthusian legacy apparent in a range of nineteenth-century literary and extra-literary writings.

Eliot's novel *Silas Marner* appears, at first glance, an agonizingly precious tale of redemption wherein the vivacity of innocent childhood serves to revive the awkward ossifications of age. *Silas Marner* is therefore frequently cited as an exemplar of Eliot's expansive organicist worldview, a "ubiquitous" ideal throughout the Victorian period associated with "harmonious cultural integration and gradual social development" (Shuttleworth, *Eliot* x). A plot summary supports this impression. Sometime in the late eighteenth century, Silas Marner arrives in the rural village of Raveloe as an exile from Lantern Yard, having been framed for theft. Despite his debilitating loneliness, Silas's sense of alienation is somewhat offset by the gold he earns as a linen weaver. One winter evening fifteen years after his arrival, he is devastated to discover that his fortune has been stolen. Weeks later, the still-bereft Silas opens his cottage door and falls into a cataleptic trance; at this moment a toddler enters (her opium-addicted mother has perished in the snow under a nearby furze-bush) and, when Silas regains consciousness, he initially mistakes the golden-haired child for his lost gold. To the villagers' surprise, Silas immediately adopts Eppie as his daughter and, in the process of raising her, forges the social bonds with Raveloe that he once refused. Sixteen years pass (the most overt of several resonances with Shakespeare's *The Winter's Tale*, a work that also sees the restoration of harmonious relations between old and young), until the near-simultaneous discovery of Silas's long-lost fortune and Eppie's well-bred parentage. In spite of the offer she receives to lead the comfortable life of a gentry-woman, Eppie refuses to abandon Silas, her "little old daddy," and chooses instead to marry the conscientious young gardener whom she has loved since childhood (*SM* 199). The novel ends with a Voltairean flourish as the "four united people"—Silas, Eppie, Aaron, and his mother, Dolly—return from the wedding to live out their days amidst a budding garden (244).

Looking aslant at Eliot's shortest novel, however, we can take *Silas Marner*'s preoccupation with the inevitability of change, diminution, and decay as a manifold meditation on waste and repair. In an 1861 letter to John Blackwood, George Eliot wrote of her new novel, "I don't wonder at your finding my story, as far as you have read it, rather somber: indeed, I should not have believed that any one would have been interested in it but myself (since Wordsworth is dead) if Mr. Lewes had not been strongly arrested by it" (*ELL* 401). The centrality of waste and repair to *The Physiology of Common Life* perhaps gives some indication as to why Lewes would be so "arrested" by Eliot's tale of an aging weaver. *Silas Marner* speaks to the complex texture of Victorian ideas around human aging by employing, and elaborating upon, this Lewesian principle: first, by way of characters that are themselves composites of youth and age, and second, by imagining a socialized ethos that reflects this embodied intergenerationality. Whereas the Romantic youth model viewed youth as separate from and essentially antagonistic to older age, Eliot's uptake of waste and repair suggests how its intrinsic mixedness might be reiterated as the association of "Old and Young" (notably, the title of book II of *Middlemarch*). Where Lewes focuses on the interior physiological simultaneity of these forces, however, Eliot's imagination transmutes them into the collective context. Bodily wasting presents an opportunity for both individual and social repair.

From the decline of rural industry and skills to the climactic draining of the Stone-Pits, Lewes's startling "Life is waste" echoes throughout *Silas Marner* as an underpinning reality principle. Consider the novel's very first sentence:

> In the days when the spinning-wheels hummed busily in the farmhouses—and even great ladies, clothed in silk and thread-lace, had their toy spinning-wheels of polished oak—there might be seen in districts far away among the lanes, or deep in the bosom of the hills, certain pallid undersized men, who, by the side of the brawny country-folk, looked like the remnants of a disinherited race. (*SM* 51)

Eliot immediately establishes this pastoral world as triply diminished: first, by the temporal distance imposed by the receding historical reality of vital rural life ("in the days when . . ."), reduced again by the perspectival effects of the "deep" and "far away" environs of Raveloe, and finally, by the bodily declension of certain "pallid undersized . . . remnants of a disinherited race." Indeed, the "remnant" functions variously throughout this passage. First rings the epithet ("a small portion, a fragment, a scrap" [*OED*]) that describes the humbled remains of a life form scarcely animated by vital juices. The human fragment under consideration is, of course, Silas Marner, whose wasted remains serve to distinguish the strapping healthfulness of rural life from the insalubrious conditions of the city. This is also an insult considered at some length by Daniel Deronda, whose assessment of Grandcourt as the "remnant of a human being" is couched within a longer meditation on the latter's "worn out . . . natural healthy interest in things" (whereas the love of a young girl will help reanimate Marner, Grandcourt remains unmoved by Gwendolen's frolics) (*DD* 334). As opposed to Grandcourt's individualized atrophy, in *Silas Marner* there is a whiff of the gothic in this residual being's belonging to a "disinherited race," a biologized inflection of the remnant as "a small remaining number of people" (*OED*), whose creeping representatives seem to signal the extinction of a family or genus. *Silas Marner*'s early diminutions immediately weave together character, setting, and form. The remnant functions as a means of viewing not only persons or characters, but also the fictional world of the proximal past, as iterations of waste and repair.

However, to "look like" the remnant does not necessarily entail one's imminent dissolution. As Eliot's reader would already know, the blanched weaver who arrives from the industrializing "North'ard" also signifies the end of the smaller-scale labors of the spinning-wheel (*SM* 54). Thus the "great ladies" and the "brawny country-folk," despite their current social and corporeal prosperity, also amount to ominous remnants of their own kind. Such bodies unwittingly imitate this transitional moment between spinning and weaving, living fragments soon to be snipped away from the social fabric—like the "end of a piece of cloth" (*OED*), or a piece of ornamental thread-lace—by the machinations of historical progress. These great figures will be disinherited by history soon enough, and by novel's end the march of industrialization helps weaving toward extinction as well ("[Silas] had nothing but what he worked for week by week, and when the weaving was going down too—for these days was less and less flax spun—and Master Marner was none so young" [*SM* 200]). The various remnants that populate the novel's opening scene are at once the last of their species and relics preserved by Eliot's fictional exercise. Decline—historical, social, and bodily—looms large in this pastoral network by drawing attention to the remnant's dual nature.

Great ladies on spinning wheels also recall the Greek mythological image of the three Fates (Moirae), commonly represented as ancient, misshapen (arthritic?) women charged with apportioning the lifespan of mortals. As Milton describes in *Lycidas,* the thread of life was often imagined as spun, measured, and inevitably cut ("Comes the blind Fury with th'abhorred shears, / And slits the thin-spun life" [75–76]), and the immediacy of Eliot's allusion works to signify the linkage of Marner's corporeal fate with the evocatively textual basis of his labour itself ("the *tale* of the cloth he wove" [*SM* 55, emphasis added]). While this mythological resonance almost certainly informs *Silas Marner*'s status as a kind of "legendary tale" (*ELL* 401), together with the opening sentence's perspectival diminutions it also directs attention to the eponymous protagonist's aging body. Early on we read that the weaver "was so withered and yellow, that, though he was not yet forty, the children always called him 'Old Master Marner'" (*SM* 69). This inconsistency in chronological and apparent age has mystified not only the hapless residents of Raveloe, but generations of scholars and illustrators as well. The Lewesian leitmotif of waste and repair helps untease these ideas by speaking, for example, to the interwoven nature of youth and age in this novel—or, as we shall see, the consequences associated with the refusal or inability to forge such linkages in the collective intergenerational context. The contradictory nature of the remnant is one thread of continuity between this range of hitherto unlinked assessments of *Silas Marner*.

Following his wrongful exile from Lantern Yard, Silas distinctly calls to mind Lewes's industrious weaver, wasting as he neglects "the calls of hunger" (64) and "drawing less and less for his own wants, trying to solve the problem of keeping himself strong enough to work sixteen hours a day on as small an outlay as possible" (67). Like Lewes's physiological spendthrift, Silas's unremitting labors are directed toward animating his monetary savings rather than his own life. Moreover, Silas's wasting of his living fabric is matched by the "superfluous" quantity of linen he produces for "homesteads . . . where women seemed to be laying up a stock of linen for the life to come" (64). We learn that Silas's economic wealth comes at the direct expense of his physical health; before meeting Eppie, and especially after the loss of his gold, Silas is described as a "pale thin figure" (106), a "poor mushed creatur" [sic] (130), one whose life is "reduce[d] to the unquestioning activity of a spinning insect" (64–65). As we read of "the bent, tread-mill attitude of the weaver" (52), Silas's gradual ossification also embodies the growing imbalance of waste, leaning as it is toward rigidity rather than movement. Like Wordsworth's leech-gatherer, Silas's physical isolation serves to dislodge him from the organic realm, so much so that his body begins to resemble the stone-pits in which he lives. "[Y]ear after year, Silas Marner had lived in this solitude, his guineas rising in the iron pot, and his life narrowing and hardening itself more and more into a mere pulsation of desire and satisfaction that had no relation to any other being" (*SM* 68). Silas wastes, it seems, as a result of his extraction from the dyadic relationships he once enjoyed in Lantern Yard—be it with his former fiancée, Sarah, or his best friend, William Dane, with whom he was known as "David and Jonathan" (*SM* 57). Silas's traumatic solidification is textually inscribed in Eliot's polysyndetic listing of airless pairs ("narrowing and hardening . . . more and more . . . desire and satisfaction").

Under these conditions, it is not surprising that readers have unhesitatingly referred to Silas as a "miser," especially given his appearance of older age.[19] Simon J. James, for example, argues that "Eliot's miser Silas Marner has been desocialized by his inability to make the hermeneutic leap from money's material existence to its intended social function," an observation consistent with the essentially static symbolic properties of the miser figure since the classical period (11). Besides, there remains the sense that older age is itself a kind of grasping condition motivated by the diminutions of the aging process, as reflected in literary and medical representations of older age throughout the nineteenth century. Wordsworth, again:

> Thus fares it still in our decay:
> And yet the wiser mind
> Mourns less for what Age takes away,
> Than what it leaves behind. ("The Fountain," 33–36)

The parsimonious hand of age splits, parses, and divides the balance of life from its senescent remainder, a sentiment voiced in Wordsworth's "The Fountain" (1800) and one that resurfaces in George Day's 1849 *A Practical Treatise on the Domestic Management and Most Important Diseases of Advanced Life*. Day directly quotes Sir James Paget's "invaluable" *Lectures on Nutrition, Hypertrophy, and Atrophy* (1847), in which the latter explains, "[s]ome people, as they grow old, seem only to wither and dry up, sharp featured, spinous old folks, yet withal wiry and tough, clinging to life, and letting death have them . . . by small instalments slowly paid" (Day 54). Here, the older person is imagined as a species of peculiarly obstinate life, bearing spikes like an ornery cactus—rather than the ripe fruits Cicero imagines in *De Senectute*—whose lingering vigor is evinced only in its anxious grasping toward life. Of course, such formulations of bodily age appeared well before the nineteenth century (consider the elderly Milton's prudent account of how one's light is spent, or King Lear's disastrous calculation of his filial legacy). Paget conspicuously updates the customary botanical image of bodily dissipation ("withering") by integrating a physio-economic conceit that apprehends life's vital force in terms of a sort of capital, thus painting any aging human Struldbrug as a kind of physiological miser.

Certainly at the outset of Eliot's novel, Silas Marner's strange relationship to his gold could be easily understood as the kind of "clinging" life in older age Paget describes. "The light of his faith quite put out, and his affections made desolate, [Silas] had clung with all the force of his nature to his work and his money" (*SM* 92). Silas's burying of his fortune further recalls Aesop's fable of a miser who, like Silas, is entirely distraught at the theft of his gold and is chided for his failure to engage the money's circulating function. Where Aesop's tale ends at the moment of the miser's comeuppance, however, the principle of waste and repair meaningfully distinguishes Silas from other misers of English literature like Shylock (*The Merchant of Venice*), Ebenezer Balfour (*Kidnapped*), Ebenezer Scrooge (*A Christmas Carol*), or even Eliot's own Featherstone (*Middlemarch*). Although both *A Christmas Carol* and *Silas Marner* take place around Christmas and describe male workaholics whose wives-to-be have left them, Scrooge—"a squeezing, wrenching, grasping, scraping, clutching, covetous old sinner!"

(*CC* 40)—indefinitely retains his fiancée while accumulating an unending fortune. Silas, on the other hand, expresses a profound sense of bereavement at his best friend's double-pronged deceit (William frames Silas for theft in order to marry Sarah). Although Scrooge and Silas both have confrontations with children that are key to effecting their recovery, their registers could not differ more. Scrooge's nightmarish interaction with the Malthusian personifications of "Ignorance" and "Want" is profoundly gothic—from his initial confusion of the children for beasts ("I see something strange . . . Is it a foot or a claw?" [*CC* 99]), to their repulsive appearance ("wretched, abject, frightful, hideous, miserable" [*CC* 99]), to their questionable claim to be children at all ("a stale and shrivelled hand, like that of age, had pinched, and twisted them, and pulled them into shreds . . . Where angels might have sat enthroned, devils lurked, and glared out menacing" [*CC* 101]). Scrooge's conversion is facilitated by an explicitly Malthusian ephebiphobia, as the Ghost of Christmas Present warns Scrooge, "most of all beware this boy, for on his brow I see that written which is Doom" (*CC* 101). Whereas Scrooge once hoarded his money as a means of prolonging his future prospects, his epiphany is facilitated by a fear of the future only different in kind.

Scrooge's eye to the fearsome future is consistent with the miser's desire to thwart the inevitable wasting of life by relentlessly hoarding an illusory substitute: money serves as the reparative prosthesis for the wasting body. (Our own day reveals a fascinating refraction of exactly this logic, as global spending on soft-tissue fillers and neuromuscular injectables reaches the hundreds of billions: in terms of symbolic progeny, the anti-aging "industry" appears the global manufactory of the new, collective miserdom of youth.) Silas's trials, conversely, take place within a less obviously supernatural framework. His turn away from the world resembles less Bosch's allegorical "Death and the Miser" (the emblematic basis of Scrooge's or Featherstone's bed-bound crises) than Pieter Breughel the Elder's "The Misanthrope" (1568; see figure 3.1 on page 82). Considering this painting alongside *Silas Marner* seems apposite for several reasons. Eliot admired the seventeenth-century Dutch masters and her taste for these images is reflected often in her early works (for instance, in the often-cited carrot-scrapers in chapter 17 of *Adam Bede*). Furthermore, the symbolism of "The Misanthrope" distinctly recalls the first catastrophe of Silas's life, from the young pickpocket that appears in the globe capped with a Christian cross (the narrow religiosity of Lantern Yard), to the knife used in the act of cutting the misanthrope's purse (William plants Silas's knife at the scene, and Silas is described as "cut off" from his former life twice in the second chapter), to the sheepherder that

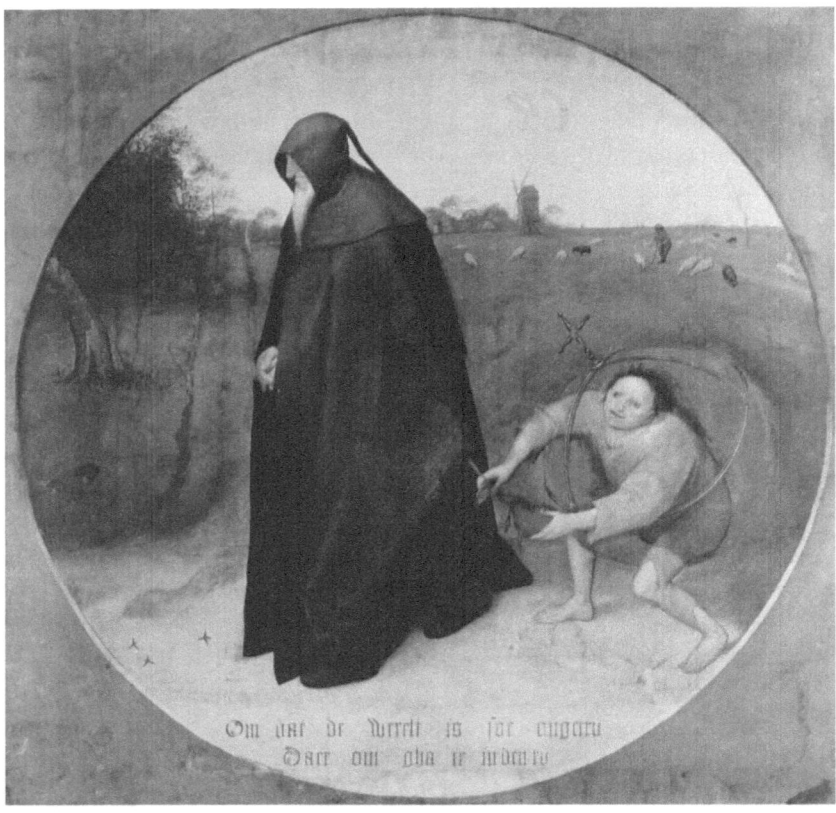

Figure 3.1. Pieter Breughel the Elder. "Misanthrop" [The Misanthrope]. Wikimedia Commons. commons.wikimedia.org/wiki/File:Pieter_Bruegel_d._%C3%84._035.jpg. Public domain.

appears in the background as a symbol of pastoral simplicity (such a figure observes the "alien-looking" weaver at the outset of *Silas Marner*). Indeed, it also recalls Silas's second catastrophe, when the yobbish Dunsey steals Silas's gold quite literally from under him. Like Breughel's misanthrope (whose Flemish legend reads, "Because the world is faithless, I am going into mourning"), and unlike the misers I've described so far, Silas has no vision of the future ("the future was all dark" [*SM* 65]). Moreover, Eliot seems at pains to reiterate that forces out of the weaver's control unjustly diminished his "withered and shrunken" life: "in reality it had been an eager life, filled with immediate purpose which fenced him in from the wide, cheerless unknown. It had been a clinging life; and though the object round which its fibres had clung was a dead disrupted thing, it satisfied the need for clinging" (*SM* 129). The pitiable image of Silas's "clinging," together with his chronic "sense of bereavement" (*SM* 190), hints at a kind of congenital, physiological instinct rather than Scrooge's squeezing and self-preserving covetousness.

Key thematic and figurative elements of *Silas Marner: The Weaver of Raveloe* therefore point toward the Lewesian vision of waste and repair described in *The Physiology of Common Life*. Eliot's choice of a weaver as her novel's protagonist (not to mention the further alliterative continuity suggested by the novel's setting, *Ravel*oe) directly gestures toward Lewes's central principle. Moreover, the multiple manifestations of Silas's strangely wandering life—from his geographical traversals, to his epilepsy, to the metempsychotic migration between animal, plant, insect, and inorganic life forms—all serve as plausible recapitulations of the dynamic fluidity of states Lewes described as fundamental to human life. However, Eliot does not merely evoke the simultaneity of waste and repair by presenting Silas as a puzzling fusion of youth and age. Instead, *Silas Marner* imagines waste and repair as a restorative social principle capable of realizing a harmonious state of intergenerational relations. Eliot recasts Lewes's physiologically intragenerational principle of waste and repair as a socializing ethic of intergenerationality: youth and age, rather than states intrinsic to the individual, become the condition of a healthy social body as well.

Tamara Silvia Wagner describes Silas's first transition as his shift from the religious faith of Lantern Yard to a "new belief in exchange-value" (86). Certainly Silas's move to Raveloe is signified by his substitution of his "sense of the Invisible" (*SM* 53) to the economic outlay of the invisible hand. However, Eliot's introduction of Eppie takes this migration one step further, as I will show, by looking to the physiological reality of the hand—so easily abstracted to signify dismal misery economics—as a fleshly cipher of the lived mutuality of waste and repair. My argument here aligns with recent studies by Peter J. Capuano and Pamela Gilbert, each of whom has demonstrated the significance of hands as a figure of speech as well as a corporeal form in the context of Victorian literature.[20] Eliot's renegotiation of generational relationships through such figurations of the hand begins, of course, with Silas's famous confusion of the newly arrived infant Eppie with his lost gold. "He felt his heart beat violently, and for a few moments he was unable to stretch out his hand and grasp the restored treasure. . . . He leaned forward at last, and stretched forth his hand; but instead of the hard coin with the familiar resisting outline, his fingers encountered soft warm curls" (*SM* 167). However, Silas presently finds himself the subject of the stranger's incarnate touch as Eppie's "small hand began to pull Marner's withered cheek with loving disfiguration" (175). This gesture recapitulates Silas's immediate sense of his urgent mutuality with the solitary infant: "it's a lone thing—and I'm a lone thing. My money's gone, I don't know where—and this is come from I don't know where" (176). Silas and Eppie are, at diverse points in their life-course, viewed as lives destined for the workhouse, and the weaver's refusal to deliver the baby to the parish takes the form of a dialogical chiasmus that links his own life to that of this alien being.

Waste and repair thus not only inform Silas's odd status as both youthful and aged, but also serve as a means of apprehending the mutuality of youth and age in terms of their social bonds. *Silas Marner*'s frequently cited allusion to the Biblical story of Lot illustrates exactly the shift I'm describing:

> In old days there were angels who came and took men by the hand and led them away from the city of destruction. We see no white-winged angels now. But yet men are led away from threatening destruction: a hand is put into theirs, which leads them forth gently toward a calm and bright land, so that they look no more backward; and the hand may be a little child's. (*SM* 190–191)

In his essay "Covenant in Hyperbole: The Disruption of Tradition in 'Michael,'" David Collings provides an extensive reading of the significance of the proximity of Lot's story to Abraham's sacrificial covenant described in Genesis 17, while Jeff Nunokawa detects in this episode nothing less than a "propaganda campaign on behalf of familial propriety" (275). Given the generational fascinations of its references—the King James Bible even cites Lot's confrontation of "old and young" in Genesis 19:4—it's clear that Eliot is working closely with a rich nexus of allusions and ideas in this crucial passage. Yet Eliot is no simple moralizer. Notice how this passage foregrounds the fleshly reality of the hand. Such "white-winged angels" are no longer—an extinct artifact of those "old days"—along with the ghastly social cataclysms they portended. In place of such celestial forms of election comes another strange visitor possessed by mortal attenuations. The passivity of the incarnate child (whose hand is "put into" another's and "leads . . . forth gently") argues for a very different model of earthly preservation than the abstractedly immortal grasp that takes and directs. Man's life, the passage intones, is not exclusively the providence of disembodied forces; for Silas, this includes the "obscure religious life" that would decide the first catastrophe of his life by drawing lots to determine his innocence or guilt (61). Waste and repair—from the vision of Lot's destruction, to the restorative possibilities of human relationships—is figured in the joint image of youth and age.

Silas is banished to live among the rubble of this past life, fittingly enough, in the Stone-Pits of Raveloe, where unbeknownst to him he will encounter yet another "young winged thin[g]" (as he himself was described in Lantern Yard) (*SM* 58). Before Eppie's arrival the weaver's hand is quite literally the architect of his life, as "Silas's hand satisfied itself with throwing the shuttle" (64). Yet the hand also functions as a sign of another kind, namely, the generational kinship relations that mark the climax of the novel sixteen years later. Childless and wishing to make their claim on Eppie, Godfrey Cass and his wife enter the weaver's cottage the night Silas's stolen gold is recovered. Hands figure prominently throughout this episode, and demonstrate how economic relationships may be starkly at odds with affective bonds. As Godfrey introduces his plan to raise Eppie as a gentry-woman, Eppie immediately moves to contact Silas ("Eppie had quietly passed her arm behind Silas's head, and let her hand rest against it caressingly: she felt him trembling violently" [229]; "Eppie took her hand from her father's head, and came forward a step" [230]; "She retreated to her father's chair again, and held him round the neck: while Silas, with a subdued sob, put up his hand to grasp hers" [230]). Silas refuses Godfrey's plans by describing his intensely somatic identification with his adopted daughter. "How'll she feel just the same for me as she does now, when we eat o' the same bit, and drink o' the same cup, and think o' the same things from one day's end to another? Just the same? that's idle talk. You'd cut us i' two" (231). Nor is Silas's logic one-sided. When the terms are put plainly to her, Eppie refuses Godfrey's offer in a now legible emblem of association. "She held Silas's hand in hers, and grasped it firmly—it was a weaver's hand, with a palm and finger-tips that were sensitive to such pressure—while she spoke with colder decision than before" (233).

Old and young holding hands: while this may strike our ears as sentimental or even maudlin, Eliot's story asserts the extent to which Eppie and Silas's lives are interwoven.[21] More than this, Eliot engages with two important and as-yet-unremarked intertexts that supplement the physiological principles Lewes describes. First: *Silas Marner*'s intergenerational gambit asks us to recall Blake's *Songs of Innocence and of Experience*, which contains several illustrations of old and young in a state of such physical mutuality.

86 ☙ The Aesthetics of Senescence

David Leon Higdon has noted Eliot's use of Blake's *Songs* as epigraphs in *Middlemarch*, arguing that there, as in Eliot's other novels, such epigraphs "are a foreshadowing of what follows, and to some degree shape, control, and condition the reader's reaction to the chapter . . . behind them is a carefully enunciated concept of form" (Higdon 131). In *Silas Marner* Blake is put to similar use, albeit imagistically. Consider Blake's personification of the human hand in plate 84 of *Jerusalem*, for example, or "London" (see figure 3.2)—the latter particularly interesting for its resonance with Silas

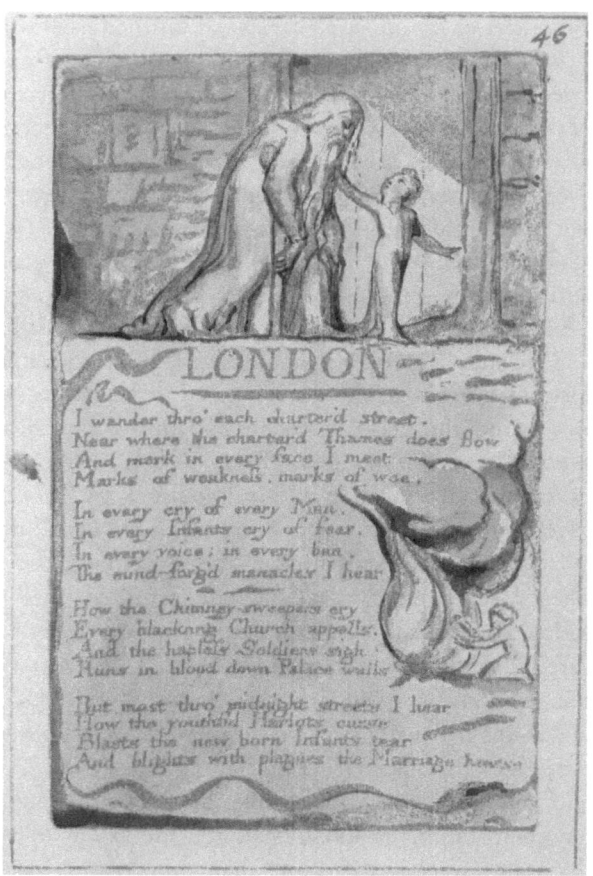

Figure 3.2. William Blake. "London." From *Songs of Innocence and of Experience: Shewing the Two Contrary States of the Human Soul* [Songs of Experience]. London, 1794. © The Trustees of the British Museum. All rights reserved.

and Eppie's walk through the chartered streets of Lantern Yard in the novel's closing pages. Likewise, the plates of "The Ecchoing Green" (see figure 3.3 on pages 88 and 89) depict an "Old John" leading the village youth homeward, as sunset parleys the end of the day's amusements:

> Like birds in their nest
> Are ready for rest:
> And sport no more seen
> On the darkening Green. (Blake, *Songs* 27–30)

"The Ecchoing Green" mutually implicates old and young in the activity of waste and repair, as the children's lively expenditures in plate 1 are pendant with their blithe fatigue in plate 2. Blake's cyclical imagery figures strongly in these illustrations; while Old John rests in the midst of the children's play in the first plate, plate 2 portrays his active lead via the children's supplicating gestures and his extended arm pointing homeward at the day's end. This social positioning of the aged is significant for how it implicates not only older age and youth, but male and female also: just as Old John is depicted among three mothers, so is Silas referred to as a kind of compound parent to Eppie.

Eliot's narrative strongly evokes yet another ancient tale of loss and restoration. In Plato's *Symposium*, Aristophanes offers a fable to explain the purpose of and drive behind erotic love, particularly the sense of completeness or wholeness that is generated by finding one's soul mate. Aristophanes tells the story of an original human nature, in which three sexes—man, woman, and the union of the two—were coupled to compose fantastic, eight-limbed, dyadic human beings. Afraid of these beings' awesome strength, Zeus decides to cut each being in half, leaving the belly-button as the sole relic of this primeval state of oneness:

> After the division the two parts of man, each desiring his other half, came together, and throwing their arms about one another, entwined in mutual embraces, longing to grow into one, they began to die from hunger and self-neglect, because they did not like to do anything apart; and when one of the halves died and the other survived, the survivor sought another mate, man or woman as we call them,—being the sections of entire men or women,—and clung to that. (Plato 522)

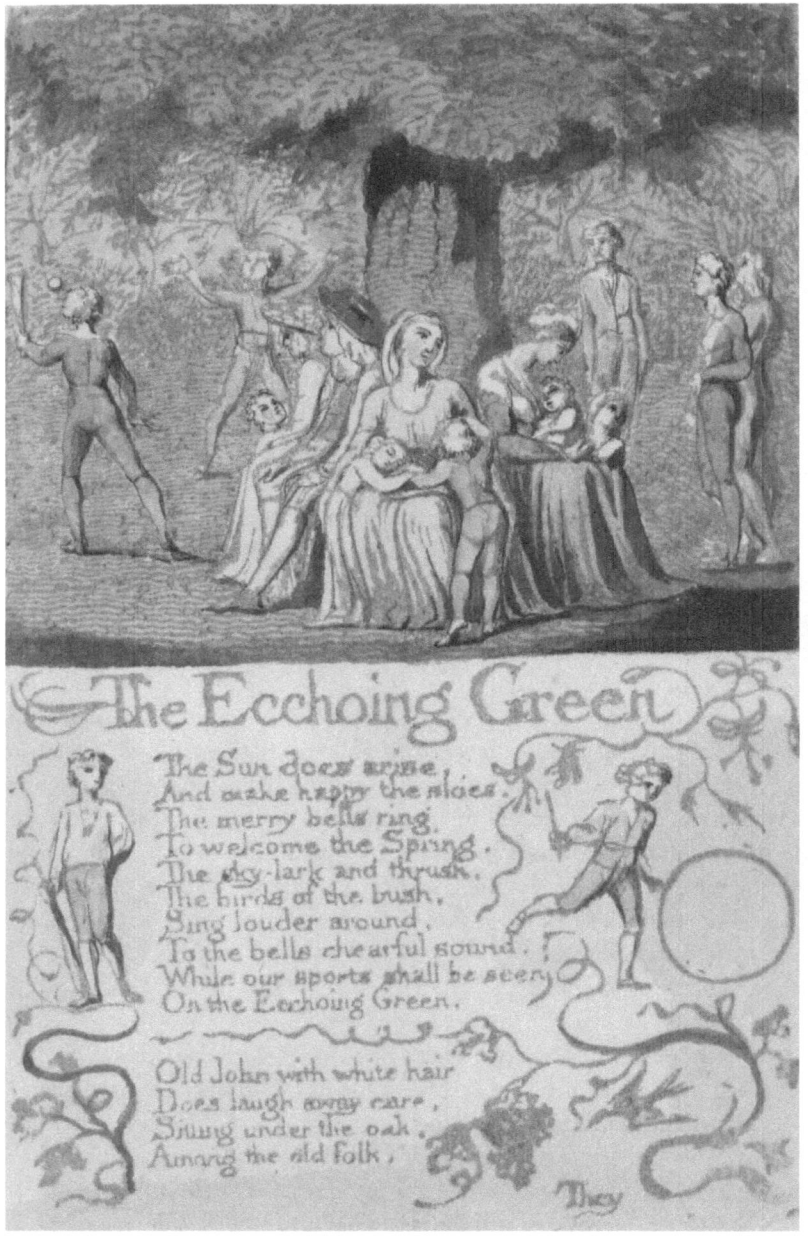

Figure 3.3. William Blake. "The Ecchoing Green" [recto, Plate 1, and verso, Plate 2]. From *Songs of Innocence and of Experience: Shewing the Two Contrary States of the Human Soul* [Songs of Innocence]. London, 1789. © The Trustees of the British Museum. All rights reserved.

They laugh at our play,
And soon they all say.
Such such were the joys.
When we all girls & boys,
In our youth time were seen,
On the Ecchoing Green.

Till the little ones weary
No more can be merry
The sun does descend,
And our sports have an end:
Round the laps of their mothers,
Many sisters and brothers,
Like birds in their nest,
Are ready for rest:
And sport no more seen,
On the darkening Green.

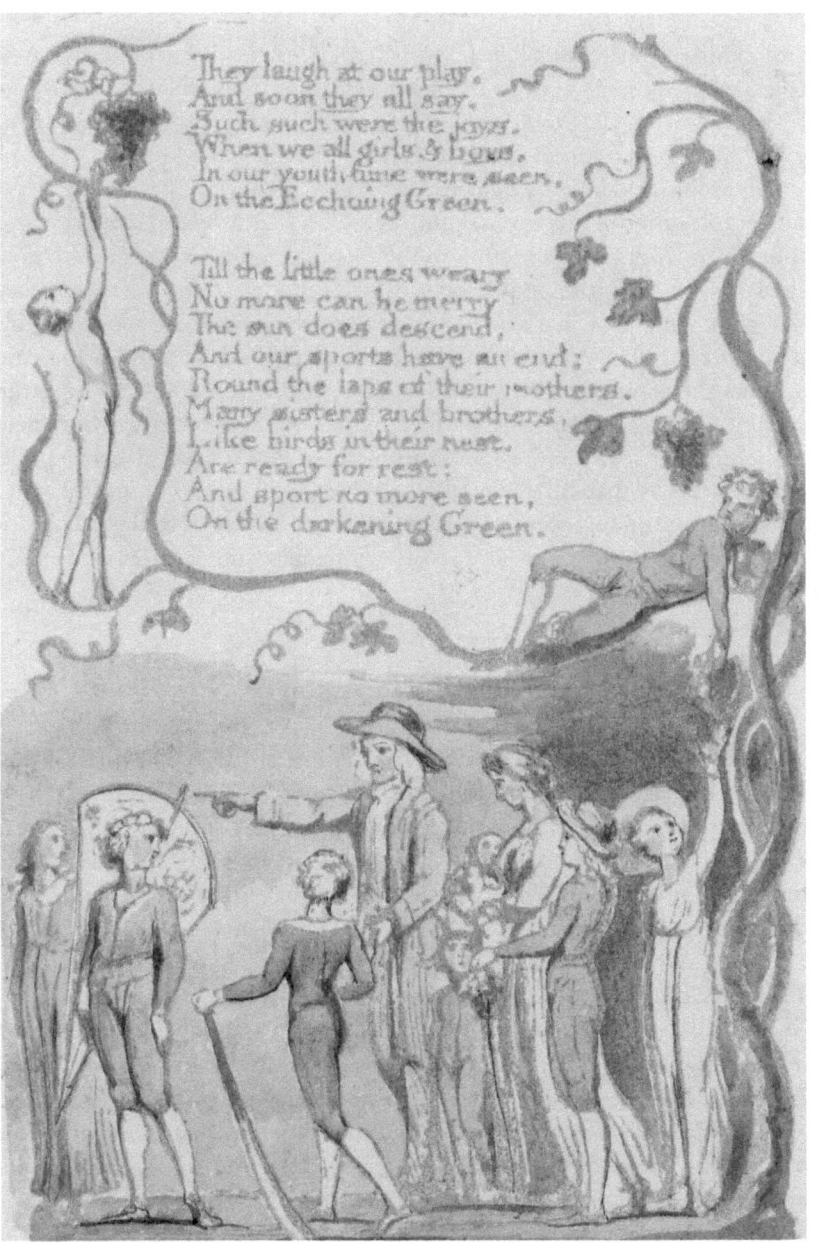

Eliot similarly imagines a life in which what has been cut in two can be joined again. At several points the novel reflects on Silas's duality of gendered attributes—from his weaving, to his "natural" ability for childcare, to his being "both father and mother" to Eppie—signaling the kind of abundant hermaphroditic ideal Aristophanes describes. This cleavage of the self is apparent in other motifs throughout the novel, hence *Silas Marner*'s formulation of epilepsy as a wandering soul ("the thief must have come and gone while I was not in the body, but out of the body" [60]; or, "there might be such a thing as a man's soul being loose from his body, and going out and in, like a bird out of its nest and back" [55]). Whereas Aristophanes imagines the completion of the self in terms of the cleft and clinging nature of erotic love, Eliot imagines another species of shared life in which what has been cut in two can be joined again. Like Plato's severed beings, Eliot seeks to repair—that is, by literally *re-pairing*—the severed states of youth and age: an intriguing gambit, not unlike Mary Shelley's conclusions in *The Last Man*, that hints at the advantages of intergenerational over other social bonds, including the sexual.

Living with Aging

Decades in advance of Merleau-Ponty's assertion of the body-subject, Eliot's gestural language of the hand functions as an alternative kind of speech—a somatic substratum to language that undergirds these scenes of intergenerational contact. Whereas the Romantic youth model viewed youth as separate from or even antagonistic to older age, Eliot's novel indicates the depth to which waste and repair is embedded in her work—not just in *Silas Marner*, but also, I contend, in Eliot's authorial ethos as it responds to the frailties of Romanticism and the legacy of its youth model.

Silas is not the only character that lives in a state of intergenerational simultaneity. Eppie recapitulates this pattern as well. She is a Romantic child who becomes in Eliot's story an anachronistic (that is, "aged" in a literary-historical sense) figure of youth, one who, like Silas the weaver, lives on long after her time has come and gone. In a letter to John Blackwood shortly before *Silas Marner* was published, Eliot made a last-minute request to include lines 146–148 of Wordsworth's "Michael: A Pastoral Poem" (1800) as an epigraph to her rapidly composed novel. She wondered, however, whether the "motto . . . indicates the story too distinctly?" (Haight 385). Eliot does not elaborate on how this excerpt—

> A child, more than all other gifts
> That earth can offer to declining man,
> Brings hope with it, and forward-looking thoughts ("Michael,"
>   144–146)

—might "too distinctly" marshal the reader, especially given the profound differences that exist between *Silas Marner* and its literary forebear. Beyond the obvious differences in form (poem/novel), the aged Michael is unusually strong, while Silas is unusually frail; Michael's son, Luke, abandons his elderly parents, while Eppie insists on remaining with Silas; whereas "Michael" must be read as a failure of intergenerational bonding, Silas Marner's is, on the whole, a successful one. What I find interesting is that it is through both Eppie's character—and her textual avatar, the *epi*-graph—that Eliot revises the outcome of "Michael" to repair Wordsworth's tragedy of failed generational relations.

In the context of Wordsworth's poem, lines 146–148 set up the tragic contrast between Michael's hopes for his newborn son and their eventual outcome. As a young man, Luke finds himself tasked with the duty to "repair"—Wordsworth's word—the financial losses incurred by a distant relative (252). Before he leaves, Michael insists that Luke erect a concrete sign of his filial bonds, joining "old and young"—a phrase that Wordsworth uses twice in this narrative poem—in the form of a stone sheepfold. The task is never completed, and the unrepaired rubble stands forward only as an ironic realization of Michael's wish that "a covenant / Twill be between us" (414–415): "between" denoting here an obstruction rather than a common link (as in, the covenant will stand between us). As in *Silas Marner*, the movement of hands is crucial at the poem's climactic moment, but the mutuality that constantly characterizes Silas and Eppie's relationship is nowhere to be found. Luke simply follows the directions implied by his father's hand, which "point[s] to the stones" (303) Michael intends to make a sign of Luke's covenant: "Lay now the corner-stone / As I requested" (403–404). The covenant is doomed, not so much because "Michael and Luke cannot quite symbolize their affections" (as Collings has argued, "Covenant" 562), but because this concretization of relations is so unilaterally and, generationally speaking, unidirectionally constructed. Abandoned by Luke, predeceased by his wife, the elderly Michael dies and the poem ends, but not before the reader learns that his cottage has been ploughed over as he had foretold: wasted, readers are told, by "a stranger's hand" (231, 477).

The pastoral tragedy of "Michael" seems an inauspicious starting point for Eliot's novel. But by selecting only the lines she does, Eliot recasts Wordsworth's words as newly forward-looking. Forward-looking in the hopeful sense, certainly, as the novel ends with Silas, Eppie, and her new husband returning to their cottage, a happy retreat from the twin realities of population and monetary capitalism that now haunt Lantern Yard. Yet the novel may be forward-looking in a less sentimental, perhaps less dishonest sense too, since by the end of *Silas Marner* incarnate realities do prevail. Despite the wonder of Marner's improved eyesight and social integration, we are told that "in everything else one sees signs of a frame much enfeebled by the lapse of . . . sixteen years" (*SM* 120). Marner's indisputable bodily frailty effectively moderates the received view of *Silas Marner* as a sentimental fable, a zero-sum narrative in which monetary loss is compensated for by gains in other quarters. Without turning away from the necessary loss in later life—as Wordsworth himself emphasized just two lines after those Eliot chose for her epigraph—Eliot also speaks to the inexorability of old age, to a time when the future prospects of "declining man . . . / By tendency of nature *needs must* fail" (Wordsworth, "Michael" 148–150, emphasis added). Marner's advice to Eppie articulates this inevitability using the very terms found in these lines but with differing import: "things will change, whether we like it or not; things won't go on for a long while just as they are and no difference. I shall get older and helplesser, and . . . when I look for'ard to that, I like to think as you'd have somebody else besides me" (*SM* 130). Marner's forward-looking thoughts are of Eppie's continuing happiness, but framed within the consciousness of his own compulsory finitude: an affirmation of pathos and vulnerability that is devoid of mere sentiment and effected by the inevitable passage of time on the body. Again, Eppie takes hold of Silas's arm in a powerful figure of living alongside aging.

U.C. Knoepflmacher has called Eliot a "continuator" of Romanticism (16), and *Silas Marner* in part employs "Michael" as a means of signaling its Victorian response to "frail" Romanticism (as defined in the previous chapter). Through the author's hand, Eliot repairs her work with the literary remains of her predecessors: an epoch that, as Keats's "Ode on a Grecian Urn" preordained, was destined for time's own wasting process. Comparable portraits of waste and repair are evident elsewhere in Eliot's fiction, including the other half of *Silas Marner*'s double plot, as well as *Middlemarch* and *Daniel Deronda*. A brief comparison of Silas's narrative with that of Godfrey Cass (Eppie's secret father) reveals a distinction between those who embrace the dynamic condition of waste and repair and those who refuse such simultaneity of age states. Godfrey's refusal to live with the simultaneity of youth and age mirrors that of his father, Squire Cass, in their shared willingness to disinherit their offspring. Sixteen years later, Godfrey returns to Silas's cottage, arguably to repair the losses incurred by his refusal to acknowledge Eppie. The first paragraph of part II takes time to anatomize the ways in which Godfrey has "lost the indefinable look of youth—a loss which is marked even when the eye is undulled and the wrinkles are not yet come" (*SM* 195); Godfrey too is a kind of declining man. Like Richard's lament in Shakespeare's *The Tragedy of King Richard the Second*—"I wasted time, and now doth time waste me" (5.5.49)—in the face of Eppie and Silas's striking and embodied mutuality Godfrey is quickly disabused of his coarse reduction of bodies to the capital they represent. Where Squire Cass compulsively wastes, Nancy obsessively preserves; both instantiate not only a failure to live with aging, but, crucially, a failure to thrive, as evinced by the dying away of the Casses' title, the partitioning of their land, and Nancy's unwavering refusal to adopt despite her desire for children. Squire Cass, the unweaver of Raveloe: indeed, the Casses live according to their name, taken from the Latin *quassāre* (to dash or break in pieces) and *cassus* (empty, void, vain), from which derived the English verb meaning to make "void" or "annul" and "to discharge," "dismiss; disband, cashier." As Godfrey and Nancy return empty-handed to the Red House, he concludes, "there's debts we can't pay like money debts, by paying extra for the years that have slipped by" (*SM* 236). Eliot ensures that Godfrey's utterance occurs following the first and only time he "put[s] out his hand" to his wife (*SM* 235).

Eliot's Lewesian vision of waste and repair is also evinced more generally in her later novels. In *Middlemarch*, allusions to Blakean images of embodied youth and age occur throughout. For example, the Shelleyan Will Ladislaw is delighted to accompany the aged Miss Noble on her daily errands ("it was one of his oddities to escort when he met her in the street with her little basket, giving her his arm in the eyes of the town, and insisting on going with her to pay some call" [*MM* 422]), a fact recounted with conspicuous emphasis by Lydgate to Dorothea: "you know Ladislaw's look—a sort of Daphnis in coat and waistcoat; and this little old maid reaching up to his arm—they looked like a couple dropped out of a romantic comedy" (453). Will, however, is the exception in *Middlemarch*, a novel that reads as a study not only of provincial life, but also of persons unable to live comfortably among the simultaneity of youth and age. Fred Vincy's interaction with Featherstone constructs a tableau similar to that of Will and Miss Noble, but the narrator's interior perspective paints a very different image:

> Fred, in spite of his irritation, had kindness enough in him to be a little sorry for the unloved, unvenerated old man, who with his dropsical legs looked more than usually pitiable in walking. While giving his arm, he thought that he should not himself like to be an old fellow with his constitution breaking up; and he waited good-temperedly, first before the window to hear the wonted remarks about the guinea-fowls and the weather-cock, and then before the scanty book-shelves. (99)

The unloved Featherstone exemplifies the miser described earlier, one who compensates for the wasting of bodily strength with financial hoarding. The antipathy with which Fred beholds the aged man further serves to unstring the constitutive threads of youth and age by regarding Featherstone as an increasingly abject being ("he should not himself like to be an old fellow"). In fact, Fred's behavior reads as a milder rendering of Alice's encounter with the grotesquely sexualized Duchess in Carroll's *Alice's Adventures in Wonderland* (1865), a novel whose aging female characters, Teresa Mangum observes, "are rendered excessive, absurd, repugnant" ("Little Women" 73). In contrast to Eppie and Silas's mutuality of generational relations, Fred does little to forge meaningful contact with this "unloved, unvenerated old man." Where Eppie fiercely asserts the strength of her bonds with Silas, Fred's interior loathing reflects the emptiness of his limp intergenerational gesture.

The two poles of *Middlemarch*'s intergenerational gambit are indicated by the titles of book II ("Old and Young") and book V ("The Dead Hand"), the former a register of the possibility of mutual intergenerational relations, the latter of their division. Fred Vincy's interaction with Featherstone occurs over both registers: Fred attends to the old man under the guise of altruistic assistance and with the vulgar hope that Featherstone will rescue him from his debts. Featherstone, perhaps cognizant of Fred's clumsy charade, avenges his mortality by cutting Fred out of his will. We see the futility of Fred and Featherstone's interaction reiterated in Dorothea's marriage to Casaubon (*Cass*-aubon), in which distinct but similarly empty fictions interrupt the possibility of a successful intergenerational coupling. The following passage is one of several in *Middlemarch* wherein Dorothea and Casaubon's mutual failure to live with waste and repair is reflected in a recognizable suite of limbic imagery:

> [Casaubon's] glance in reply to hers was so chill that she felt her timidity increased; yet she turned and passed her hand through his arm.

> Mr. Casaubon kept his hands behind him and allowed her pliant arm to cling with difficulty against his rigid arm.
>
> There was something horrible to Dorothea in the sensation which this unresponsive hardness inflicted on her. That is a strong word, but not too strong: it is in these acts called trivialities that the seeds of joy are forever wasted, until men and women look round with haggard faces at the devastation their own waste has made. . . . (388)

Casaubon's "unresponsive hardness," Featherstone and Stone Court, the volcanic rockiness of Squire Cass, even the devastated rubble of Godfrey and Nancy's happiness: it is as if the refusal to acknowledge the composite nature of life as an ongoing process of waste and repair its itself a form of miserliness, hence the conspicuous association of stony wasting with Eliot's figures of failed intergenerationality. From Aesop's miser, who is told to bury a stone in place of his gold, to the several Ebenezers that populate the Victorian novel, the aged miser is rock personified. Casaubon's pathological rigidity is thus as significant an image as his aridity, denoting as it does his refusal for any sort of collective endeavor: be it intellectual, erotic, or intergenerational. Unlike Silas, Casaubon—indeed, in large part Dorothea as well—remains a "strange creatur[e]" (190) in whom waste and repair, and the physiological corollaries they imply, are destined to remain incommensurate.

And so we return to the geological underpinnings of waste and repair, which provide Eliot with a means of thinking through relationships to the past in terms of natural catastrophes. The dynamic nature of geological history, as Lyell, Lewes, and Darwin all observe, is both conservative and destructive. The theft of Silas's gold, for instance, makes his subsequent earnings "as irrelevant as stones brought to complete a house suddenly buried by an earthquake" (*SM* 130). Perhaps this is why chapter 55 of *Middlemarch* meditates on age-inflected meanings of hope via the image of geological cataclysm:

> If youth is the season of hope, it is often so only in the sense that our elders are hopeful about us; for no age is so apt as youth to think its emotions, partings, and resolves are the last of their kind. Each crisis seems final, simply because it is new. We are told that the oldest inhabitants of Peru do not cease to be agitated by the earthquakes, but they probably see beyond each shock, and reflect that there are plenty more to come. (*MM* 498)

This passage speaks to the importance of age identity to the perspectival narrative structure of Eliot's novel. For when the narrator states that youth is only hopeful insofar as "our elders are hopeful about us," the first-person plural subject implies that both the narrator and the reader form part of such a cohort. The agedness of this "we" is strangely fluid here; in three sentences the narrator negotiates both an association and disassociation with the youth whom she addresses. The Peruvian digression—a surprising because exotic locale, and one mentioned earlier by Brooke in his fruitlessly wandering political speech—seems a necessary means of chiding youth's fatalistic self-centeredness of perspective, a catastrophic outlook that is apt to view newness as a final sort of crisis—as if every youth understood themselves to be a Lionel Verney, as did Shelley while writing *The Last Man*.[22] The reader of Eliot's novel must learn to live with aging if only because it is in the nature of the genre, as Bakhtin writes, that "time becomes, in effect, palpable and visible" (250). Ultimately, Eliot's continuation of frail Romanticism and its metaphors of youth—be it the Romantic child Eppie or the Shelleyan figure of Will—reads as a kind of authorial effort to live with thoroughly anachronistic ruins of literary Romanticism itself.

Eliot's interest in the social ethos of intergenerationality extends to her final novel, *Daniel Deronda*, most notably in Daniel's interaction with his birth mother. At the novel's climax, Princess Halm-Eberstein finds herself reluctantly reunited with the son she gave up for adoption decades earlier. The embodied limbic images throughout this passage recall Eppie's clinging to Silas, but with a suite of irreconcilable differences introduced by gender:

> 'Let me look at your hand again: the hand with the ring on. It was your father's ring.'
>
> [Daniel] drew his chair nearer to her and gave her his hand. We know what kind of hand it was: her own, very much smaller, was of the same type. As he felt the smaller hand holding his, as he saw nearer to him the face that held the likeness of his own, aged not by time but by intensity, the strong bent of his nature towards a reverential tenderness asserted itself above every other impression, and in his most fervent tone he said—
>
> 'Mother! take us all into your heart—the living and the dead. Forgive everything that hurts you in the past. Take my affection.'
>
> She looked at him admiringly rather than lovingly, then kissed him on the brow, and saying sadly, 'I reject nothing, but

I have nothing to give,' she released his hand and sank back on her cushions. (*DD* 525)

Like Dorothea with Casaubon, Daniel imagines a spontaneous sort of reconciliation—an act of reparation, really—between old and young. Here Eliot complicates the terms of the limbic tableau she has relied on elsewhere by breaking down simple assignations of waste and repair. The Princess Halm-Eberstein gave up Daniel at birth in the name of pursuing a successful singing career, since to retain the child would have meant living with her choice of wasted talent. Daniel's extension of his hand and his moving plea present the opportunity to recuperate the loss incurred by this choice. Two competing ideas of waste are at stake here: Daniel's, of course, and his mother's—the latter, Eliot is at pains to emphasize, for whom a life dedicated to art was very much a recuperative and restorative one. Daniel's imperatives—"take us," "Forgive everything," "take my affection"—considered in tandem with the infantilized proportions of his otherwise "impressive" mother's hand, uncomfortably suggest the son's thrusting of his generational mandate onto his mother. However impressive the Princess may otherwise appear, it is as if youth has aimed to usurp its own generational demarcations in a manner that is difficult to separate from the expectations of gender. Like Eppie, the Princess rejects this offer from her "new unfamiliar" kin (*SM* 232), perhaps because she is all too aware of how she has been shrunken from a vigorously lined, impressive dowager into a being no more daunting than Daniel's unseemly because childlike wife-to-be Mirah. Daniel's mother is remarkably candid in her assessment of the wasting potential of restoring her filial dealings. Cordelia's seismic refusal in *King Lear* echoes loudly in the Princess's rejection and offer of "nothing," a complex symptom of maternal lack from which Daniel is "repulsed" (*DD* 526). Later she is described as "a sorceress who would stretch forth her wonderful hand and arm to mix youth-potions for others, but scorned to mix them for herself, having had enough of youth" (*DD* 547). Giving up Daniel for adoption was a symptom of her weariness of youth and the children it generates, and now, decades later, she remains just as skeptical of the reparations youth so assuredly announces. As Malthus's *Essay* asserted decades earlier, youth itself may invite a swathe of wasting. The Princess implies that the social ethics of repair reaches far beyond transactional relationships, as Godfrey Cass was to discover in *Silas Marner*. Eliot's portrait of the Princess Halm-Eberstein is remarkable for the way the gendered implications of living with aging are staged, challenged, and ultimately refused, to a degree witnessed nowhere else in Eliot's oeuvre, and perhaps in the Victorian novel.

It is merely a coincidence that 1861 marked the year of *Silas Marner*'s publication and, eight months later, the onset of Victoria's widowhood following Albert's death at age 42. However, we might look to this collision of history and literature as a means of imagining how, and when, the Victorian period crystallized its associations with older age. The "aging" of certain Romantic precursors, Wordsworth especially, became a common obsolescing tactic among Victorian writers as a means of announcing one's present artistic fitness. Besides the well-known critiques leveled by Charles Dickens in *Bleak House* and Wilkie Collins's *Woman in White*, Lewis Carroll's 1856 "Upon the Lonely Moor" (revisited and revised for *Alice's Adventures in Wonderland* as "Haddock's Eyes") takes the leech-gatherer of "Resolution and Independence" as the rapacious incarnation of Wordsworth's own archaic nonsense: a pattern of satire Carroll repeated in the didactic doggerel of "Father William" (itself a spoof of Wordsworth's Poet Laureate predecessor, Robert Southey's "The Old Man's Comforts and How He Gained Them" [1799]). Sobriety prevailed in Robert Browning, who confessed in "Pauline" (1833) that although Wordsworth had been a tremendous influence in his youth, it was necessary to put aside childish things (alas for Percy Shelley, whom Browning similarly sent away). This age-based authorly self-fashioning provides a distinctly Victorian model of inheritance whose emphases diverge from the murderous inclinations of what Harold Bloom has called the "anxiety of influence."

Eliot is remarkable for her restoration—we might almost say adoption—of such abjected Romanticism, a period that, as Keats's "Ode on a Grecian Urn" preordained, was destined for a kind of wasting. The author's hand, Eliot's especially, works as a figure of waste and repair, as her meditation on writing in the midst of *Middlemarch* makes clear. Quoting from an earlier lyrical meditation on an urn (of all things), Thomas Browne's *Hydriotaphia, or Urn Burial* (1658), Eliot describes how writing restores the suspended literary imagination, like water might a dormant rotifer:

> Who shall tell what may be the effect of writing? If it happens to have been cut in stone, though it lie face down-most for ages on a forsaken beach, or "rest quietly under the drums and tramplings of many conquests," it may end by letting us into the secret of usurpations and other scandals gossiped about long empires ago. . . . As the stone which has been kicked by

generations of clowns may come by curious little links of effect under the eyes of a scholar, through whose labours it may at last fix the date of invasions and unlock religions, so a bit of ink and paper which has long been an innocent wrapping or stop-gap may at last be laid open under the one pair of eyes which have knowledge enough to turn it into the opening of a catastrophe. (*MM* 375–376)

The simultaneity of the past in the present is, of course, exactly the nature of *Silas Marner*'s relationship to its Wordsworthian forerunner and, as this chapter has argued, Eliot's relationship to Romanticism more generally. Eliot, like Eppie or even the stone-kickers described above, assembles the abandoned stones of Michael's tragedy in order to enact a twofold repair of intergenerational relations: those embodied links at stake in the fictional world of Raveloe, and then those "bit[s] of ink and paper" which Eliot's Victorian cohort had set aside.

In its portrayal of the linkage of youth and age, *Silas Marner* becomes an opportunity to point out the failure not only of Michael's intergenerational relations but of those who would waste the project of living alongside youth and age. Michael's tragedy, like that of the Romantic youth model, is not of one of omission or refusal to notice the fact of human aging. Instead, it is the mistaken notion that youth and age exist in separate spheres which underpins the cataclysmic Romantic wasting in "Michael." *Silas Marner* revises this catastrophe to argue for the essential miscegenation of youth and age, of Romanticism and Victorianism—a desirable species of ambiguity indispensable to lasting social cohesion and, from a literary-historical perspective, a means of softening the boundaries of periodization. By inventing ways to represent the complexity of life's temporal moments as an essential aspect of wholeness and integrated being, writers like George Eliot were exploring imaginative strategies for complicating the linear directives of chronological aging and the stages model of life. Yet the happy synthesis of *Silas Marner*'s nostalgic conclusion, and the healthy intergenerational hybridity Eliot envisioned, could not endure long beyond its pages. As the century wore on, intergenerational incorporation would take on a decidedly different cast, converging earlier anxieties about overpopulation with a toxic fusion of ageism and misogyny.

Chapter 4

"The Century's corpse"

Reading Senility at the *Fin de Siècle*

The final decades of the nineteenth century witnessed a growing sense of crisis concerning Europe's cultural climate and moral direction. Facing a slew of novel forms and ideas—reflected in emergent aesthetic modes such as Impressionism, decadence, and the gritty naturalism of Émile Zola—proponents and critics of modernity alike were alive to significant shifts in the goals and desires upon which Victorian culture had built its image. On the continent, Austrian critic Max Nordau was chief among the skeptics. His bestselling treatise *Degeneration* (*Entartung*, 1892–3; English trans. 1895) sermonized against those modern artists who personified the treacherously ascendant New:

> In opposition to healthy art, which they [i.e., "degenerate" artists] deride as musty and antiquated, they pretend to represent youth.... The truth is, however, that degenerates are not only not young, but that they are weirdly senile. Senile is their splenetic calumniation of the world and life; senile are their babblings, drivellings, ravings and divagations; senile their impotent appetites, and their cravings for all the stimulants of exhaustion. To be young is to hope; to be young is to love simply and naturally; to be young is to rejoice in one's own health and strength, and in that of all human beings, and of the birds of the air and the beetles in the grass; and of these qualities there is not one to be met with among the youth-simulating, decayed degenerates. (553–554)

Striking is Nordau's abrupt rumination on senility, a term whose connotation had, by this time, shifted from the neutral "belonging to, suited for or incident to old age" in the late seventeenth century toward the categorically pathological (*OED*). By the late 1800s, to be senile was not merely to be old. It was to be beheld by the observant eye as profoundly marked with decline.

Throughout *Degeneration*, health (both in bodily constitution and artistic outlook) is the product of properly directed and proportional motivations that embody the Leibnizian doctrine of *optimisme*. Art is "young" insofar as it hopes, portrays heterosexual ("simple and natural") love, and finds itself in alignment with a pastoral view of the compatibility of human and external natures (the "birds" and the "beetles")—in stark opposition to the unremittingly corruptive effects of the urban "world and life." Senility, by stark contrast, encapsulates the double coding of moral decay and the pretended simulation of youth, in another instance of the broader *fin de siècle* tendency to invoke senescence under the banner of chronic social and even evolutionary decline. The senile degenerate (Nordau would likely read such phrasing as a dim-witted redundancy) is a host of uncanny perversions, wherein the proliferative signs of excess—from the Baudelairean idiomatics of spleen to the logorrhoeic clamor of "babblings, drivellings, ravings and divagations"—serve only to mask an existential void. Such individuals are condemned, like Tantalus, to a rapacious yet barren ("impotent") species of appetite, while the "stimulants" they crave only effect further wasteful dissipation. Nordau's weirdly emphatic index apes this empty superfluity of senility, first, through its conspicuous anaphora ("Senile is . . . senile are . . . senile their"; "greisenhaft ist" and "greisenhaft ihr" in the original German), compound negations ("not only not young"), and then, by employing flamboyant multisyllabic Latinates ("splenetic calumniations," "ravings and divagations"), as lexical indicators of such pathology.[1] By contrast, youth—real youth—is evidenced in its bare simplicity. Thus Nordau's equally insistent "[t]o be young" recurs with none of those performatively excessive senile paroxysms. Instead, the universal infinitives of "to hope," "to love," and "to rejoice" hold sway over this familiar, favored and, above all, healthful attitudinal orientation toward life.

In stark contrast to the healthful synthesis of generations portrayed in George Eliot's *Silas Marner*, in the degenerate state youth and age merge in an unseemly confusion of otherwise distinct spheres. Clearly Nordau envisions a "good" species of the old (a kind of Burkean admiration of the ancient materialized in classic forms of art erroneously "deride[d] as musty and antiquated") distinct from "bad" senility (a pathological state of decay that necessarily overlaps with the sham youthfulness of degeneracy). Senility thus emerges a complex insignia in which medicalized and aesthetic values are yoked to visions of decline that extend beyond the single individual and into the temporal realm of the world to come.[2] Speaking against such agents of the paradoxical New, Nordau stormed, "They are not progress, but the most appalling reaction. They are not liberty, but the most disgraceful slavery. They are not youth and the dawn, but the most exhausted senility, the starless winter night, the grave and corruption" (556). It is not just the improper mingling of youth and older age but the contagious threat to population it implies that lies at the basis of such "senile" contaminations. Thus *Degeneration* delineates yet another permutation of a hallmark crisis in British *fin de siècle* literary writing, namely, the alarming duality of outward pretense and inward reality: be it "bunburying" in Oscar Wilde's *The Importance of Being Earnest* (1895), or the autobiographical-cum-literary fantasies of dissemblance that limn Robert Louis Stevenson's *The Strange Case of Dr Jekyll and Mr Hyde* (1886).

Given Nordau's suspicion of bodies that contradict biological or aesthetic expressions of healthy futurity, today's readers will not be surprised that such chimerical visions would implicate the homosexual male, or "invert," as the quintessentially degenerate, senile body (to be clear: I engage these terms here as they would have been used in texts of that period). The word "senility" derives from the Latin *senex* ("old man"), and the aged roué—brimming with impotent appetites and caked in cosmetics—is practically a stock character in the *fin de siècle* landscape. As literary critic Sherwood Williams observes with respect to American novelist Frank Norris's *Vandover and the Brute* (1914), "This decadent equation of perversity and senility functions as a corollary of the initial proposition that sexual perversion in general—and homosexual desire in particular—was not instinctual (not 'natural')" (718). One aspect of this corruption is the homosexual's thwarting of heteronormative temporality, which queer theorist Lee Edelman has more recently described in terms of the Western fetishization of "reproductive futurism" and the ideological investment—both personal and political—in the Child (for Edelman always an ominously capitalized figure). Such reproductive futurism is presaged by Nordau's vision of healthy art which, while taking its formal cues from the past, always casts its view toward the redemptive future. Age studies critics including Cynthia Port, Lynne Segal, and Leni Marshall have recently begun to consider how queer temporalities inflect representations and theorizations of older age and, in keeping with such critique, Mary Russo has argued against future-oriented models of progress precisely because of their antagonism toward older persons. "Hope, desire, understanding, and optimism seem ineluctably joined against the forces of the past, the backward, the unenlightened, the old. The trajectory of a lifetime, for instance, is ideologically weighted in favor of a future goal, a going forward into empty time" (Russo in Woodward, *Figuring* 21). Although Nordau's stock would fall by the end of the subsequent decade, *Degeneration* remains a quintessential text of its time, at once reflective of and a decisive influence upon major currents of late Victorian thought in Britain and Europe.

However, it is not only the homosexual male body that challenged the vigorous heteronormative temporality of Victorian reproductive futurism. Population discourse implied discomfiting linkages between the aging woman and the sterile prospects of species itself. As Margaret Cruikshank, Kathleen Woodward, and Stephen Katz have long argued, gender is an ineluctable aspect of theorizing older age, not only because of the biological reality of the climacteric but in light of twenty-first-century demographic realities. Today far more women are aging into older age, and so pathologies of aging—conditions like mild cognitive impairment and dementias including the Alzheimer type—remain disproportionately engraved upon the aged female subject.[3] With these issues in mind, this chapter situates the "Woman Question" among a nexus of anxieties linking reproductivity, gender, and visions of pathological aging at the *fin de siècle*. To do so I map what I am calling the "senile topography" of this complex cultural and historical moment in Britain, in which aging and older age emerge as topics of concern in disciplines as diverse as medicine, psychology, popular media, and literature.

Following the geological resonances of "waste and repair" discussed in chapter 3, "senile topography" is likewise a phrase drawn from physical geography. Whereas waste and repair describe the conservative principle of landmass growth (an ideal correlative to Silas and Eppie's embodied intergenerational harmony), *senile topography* describes instead "the configuration of land which prolonged degradation has reduced nearly to a base-level plain" (*OED*). As J. Hillis Miller famously argues, topographical language was crucial to nineteenth- and twentieth-century literature and philosophy, especially for the ways it linked features of landscape and their mapping to personification.[4] Within the *fin de siècle*'s cultural landscape, where pathological aging emerged as a topic of concern for multiple disciplines, I employ "senile topography" to describe the various conceptual and metaphorical gradations of anxieties concerning decline at this time. Distinct from the solitary ravings of "old, mad, blind, despised, and dying King[s]" (be they a King Lear or a George III), old age becomes an attribute of society itself. Bodily senescence thus merges with the trope of senility, and is invoked to describe those emergent species of persons deemed responsible for compromising the futurity of late Victorian life.

Where is the female body positioned within the senile topography of *fin de siècle* culture, particularly in light of that massifed body of women who refuse to participate—or were denied participation—in the hegemonic ideals of Victorian heteroreproductive futurity? The final decades of the nineteenth century witnessed an unprecedented imbrication of anxieties concerning older age, women, and the future of England, which often clustered around the changing place of women in the domestic sphere, the corroding achievements of imperialism, and a mounting dread that culture might itself be subject to the capricious whims of evolution and its shadowy counterpart, degeneration. Major debates around the "Woman Question," including the birth of the New Woman and the demographic, political, existential implications of unmarried and thus "surplus" or "odd" women, presented serious challenges to cultural constructions of temporality. This chapter traces the interdisciplinary nexus of concerns that made the "Woman Question" a discernable substratum within the *fin de siècle*'s senile topography. I first show how the demographic phenomenon of surplus women forced a major disruption of traditional views of women's life-course and temporal models. In place of a life marked by the narrative progression of matrimony and childbirth, there emerged a new, massified female subjectivity typified by its relationship to the counterfeit: a prevalent theme of *fin de siècle* literature that belied concerns regarding the authenticity of women's "age stamp" and suspect modes of textual (re)production. I then turn to George Gissing's 1893 novel *The Odd Women* to explore how Gissing engages age as a quantitative strategy with the capacity to inform—and, more often, deform—the legibility of such counterfeit women's lives, particularly in the fraught context of heterosexual domesticity. Finally, I consider what it means that similar oldening, and indeed *senilizing*, tactics are reconstituted and magnified in the broader context of *fin de siècle* British literary writing. As an iteration of the senile topography of this period, I conclude that literary engagements with counterfeit youth such as Gissing's—and the ironic, queered vision of progress they help chart—take the anti-teleological fluidity of nineteenth-century aging and its longevity narratives to their extreme conclusion.

A Woman New but Old

In his 1869 essay "Why are Women Redundant?" William Rathbone Greg asserts that "[a] state of society *so mature*, so elaborate, so highly organized as ours cannot fail to abound in painful and complicated problems" (3, emphasis added). In this now-classic statement of the demographic crisis signaled by a growing number of unmarried (thus "redundant") women at the end of the nineteenth century, Greg attributes "involuntary celibacy" among women (18) in large part to the "growing and morbid LUXURY of the age" (19). Male profligacy, along with excessive tastes that would place "weary gaieties, and joyless luxuries" ahead of the "solid and more enduring pleasures" of marriage and childrearing (28), was targeted as the source of an immanent population catastrophe and a blow to Victorian society's healthy "matur[ity]" (3). Much like Malthus in his 1798 *Essay*, Greg draws a connection between national life-course, the reproductive conditions of the state, and the excessive bodies it contains.

Such anxieties about the future of England were increasingly coded onto visions of collective fatigue, cultural stasis, and moral erosion, as Greg laments: "We are disordered, we are suffering, we are astray, because we have *gone wrong*; and our philanthropists are labouring, not to make us go backward and go right, but to make it easier and smoother to persist in wrong" (39). In contrast, then, to Malthus's celebration of the spinster, who took individual celibacy as key to national stability, the non-reproductive woman came to represent a *bona fide* threat to the mature station of Victorian life. Two decades in advance of Nordau's apocalyptic fearmongering, Greg's concern with this surplus female population takes on a spatial, temporal, and specifically age-based logic, linking maturity with the forward-looking, masculine values of progress and, conversely, Britain's current state of disorder with perversions of that progression.

Female singledom—involuntary or otherwise—thus became a symptom of cultural exhaustion signaling the accumulating infirmities of late Victorian Britain. As work by scholars like Amy Froide, Bridget Hill, and Rita Kranidis has shown, British single women had long been viewed "as an anomalous minority and . . . resented by the men whose control they had escaped" (Hill 2). Where the Victorian cult of domesticity ("separate spheres") was often invoked to describe the proper spaces of male and female conduct during this period, the single woman's anomalous life thwarted prescribed temporalities of male and female life-course. In her description of the *fin de siècle* New Woman, Patricia Murphy observes that "within a masculinised historical perspective, the female is always defined in terms of the body," that is, by a somatised temporality shaped by the limits of reproductive life (83). Working with the temporal distinctions described by Julia Kristeva—who defines male temporality as the forward-looking teleology of history ("linear time") that marches out of the past and into the promise of the future—Murphy demonstrates that in the *fin de siècle* context, gendered visions of women's time are clearly overlaid with the dynamics of *abjection* (what Kristeva defines as "what disturbs identity, system, order. What does not respect borders, positions, rules. The in-between, the ambiguous, the composite," *Powers* 4).[5] The Nordauvian imagination of senility cited earlier demonstrates that it is not only the corrosion of demarcated sexual categories but also the merging of distinct human temporal identities that produce the worst expressions of cultural degeneration. The New Woman and her fellow degenerates thus embodied a distinctively compound species in which time-honored stamps of age and gender were blurred and ambiguous.

The Victorian twinning of gender and temporality has deep roots. Take, for example, the vision of ideal womanhood described in John Ruskin's lecture "Of Queen's Gardens," published in *Sesame and Lilies* (1865), as an exemplar of the conservative model. Like Coventry Patmore's well-known narrative poem "The Angel in the House" (1854, 1862), Ruskin's essay delineates the passive, domestic terrain of heterosexual upper-middle-class womanhood distinctly from the robust activity of outdoor, masculine life: "The man's power is active, progressive, defensive. He is eminently the doer, the creator, the discoverer, the defender. His intellect is for speculation and invention; his energy for adventure, for war, and for conquest, wherever war is just, wherever conquest necessary. But the woman's power is for rule, not for battle,—and her intellect is not for invention or creation, but for sweet ordering, arrangement and decision" (Ruskin 66). For Ruskin, woman's "rule" is as much a geometric maxim or mathematical principle of conduct, which regulates, orders, and productively prunes the courageous extensions of man's inborn realm. Where men energetically reach, extend, and encounter—physically and intellectually, as we witnessed the speculative impulses of Godwin's *Political Justice*, or in Raymond's various conquests in Shelley's *The Last Man*—woman's function is to ensure the balanced abrading of excesses generated by the bold occupations of able-bodied, vigorous manhood.

Ruskinian feminine virtue possesses both material and immaterial age-related insignia. "The perfect loveliness of a woman's countenance," Ruskin writes, "can only consist in that majestic peace, which is founded in the memory of happy and useful years,—full of sweet records; and from the joining of this with that yet more majestic childishness, which is still full of change and promise;—opening always—modest at once, and bright, with hope of better things to be won, and to be bestowed. There is no old age where there is still that promise" (69). Ruskin's ideal feminine is strangely situated between the plenitude of the past (i.e., the "sweet records" of memory) and the assurance of futurity ("*still* full of change of promise," "opening always," "hope of better things") in the form of a "majestic childishness"—an odd and distinctly Victorian formulation of adult female subjectivity inflected, no doubt, by what Karen Chase has identified as the powerful and paradoxical iconography of Queen Victoria. Following Albert's death in 1861, Chase explains,

> The swift passage from wife to widow transformed the spectacle of both a girl queen and a happily domesticated matron into the unstable figure of an aged monarch desperately seeking to maintain her privilege. However, and crucially, the later images did not cancel the earlier ones. At any moment the Queen could now be figured as an innocent girl, a concerned and solicitous matron, a wise and experienced elder, or, alternatively, as an old woman either exhausted or engulfed by passions made grotesque by their intensity at her "age." (*Victorians* 154)

This fluidity of Victoria's age—and along with it, visions of bodily desire alongside political power—provided the opportunity not only for salacious gossip but for literary satire. Algernon Charles Swinburne's private drama *La Soeur de la Reine* (c. 1860–1) portrayed Wordsworth as the cumbrous seducer of a nymphomaniac widow Queen Victoria (the lady falls to the unlikely enticements of *The Excursion*), while Chase describes Alice's sudden transformative growth in Carroll's *Alice's Adventures in Wonderland,* and the petulance of both the Duchess and Queen, as symptoms of a "divided cultural fantasy" concerning Queen Victoria's body (156). More generally, the literary imagination provides an ideal means for achieving the strangely suspended temporal status Ruskin describes. Numerous majestic little womenchildren populate a range of British Victorian novels, from Eliot's *Daniel Deronda* (Mirah) to Dickens's *Little Dorrit* (Amy) or *David Copperfield* (Dora), as Claudia Nelson's work describes.

Although the longstanding image of the *Lebenstreppe* generally pictured a single male or, occasionally, one joined with female figure (see figure I.1), the symbolic array of female aging remained narrow even well into the nineteenth century. To take one but influential example, the historian and poet Agnes Strickland's "The Seven Ages of Woman" (1827) apostrophizes Shakespeare while gently chiding the androcentrism of *As You Like It*'s well-known "All the World's a Stage" speech (which I discussed in my introduction):

> Thou, whose bold genius, in so short a span,
> Marked the seven stages of the life of man;
> Yet hast omitted, in thy gifted page,
> To paint the eras of his consort's age;
> Lend me thy deathless spirit, whilst I show
> Each change of Woman's days, through weal and woe.
>   (Strickland, 1–6)

Strickland's pastiche expands Shakespeare's twenty-eight lines to 169, and motherhood ("The sweetest era of the female life, / Which makes a mother of the happy wife" [Strickland, 94–95]) emerges by far the most luminous stage of female lifecourse. Almost one-third of the poem (fifty lines) is dedicated to the period designated as "youth" (chronological age is never mentioned in the poem), and the stages describing matrimony and motherhood take up another forty-three lines (a solid quarter of the poem). This happy epoch aside, however, Strickland's "The Seven Ages of Woman" is remarkably frank about recounting the dullness associated with life before motherhood, from education, to youthful naïveté, to unrequited love, to life's mundane cruelties. Widowhood and "the last great stage" (149) are recounted with similar bluntness, and the last stanza hints at the liberating glimmers promised by the older woman's imminent return to the heavenly realm ("The feverish hopes, the fears, the cares of life, / No more oppress her with their torturing strife" [150–151]). In what life remains following motherhood:

> What now remains to show
> Of Woman's days, when all has past away
> That charmed the young, the thoughtless, and the gay
> And the fair fabric totters in decay? (138–141)

Strickland imagines that the near-ghostly woman looks to a maternal redux as a final mortal reprieve in her later days: "in her children's children tastes again / Maternal pleasure and maternal pain" (161). In place of Jaques's monolithically bleak second childhood, a second motherhood awaits for Strickland's implied reader—although it too, with its "totter[ing]," timeworn "fair fabric," reads as a feeble parody of woman's perfect age.

Strickland's poem circulated for decades after its publication, and theatrical adaptations of "The Seven Ages of Woman" were a popular form of Christmas entertainment throughout the Victorian period. However, such idealized views of the individual woman's life increasingly failed to match up with the apparent demographic reality of an aging population and increasing numbers of unmarried, unreproductive women. (Importantly, there is significant doubt by demographers as to whether women were in fact "materially or practically excessive" in relation to England's capacity to accommodate workers at this time, as Rita Kranidis and others have argued [Kranidis 27].) Regardless, if it is *motherhood* that permits the realization of Ruskinian static vision of women's majestic childishness—if it is these *roles* and not chronological age that amount to the primary aspect of female identity—then what of the woman for whom marriage and motherhood are no longer the markers of life's ages? The erosion of heteronormative ideals meant that it was no longer possible to assess female subjectivity in terms of the inevitability of matrimony and motherhood. The refiguring of women's life-course indicates that in late Victorian Britain, the breakdown of separate spheres was a crisis of temporality as much as of space.

In the place of such "womanly" women, the *fin de siècle* marked the emergence of a new female subject that disturbed the compulsory age markers of life-course. The significance of the New Woman, particularly her challenge to longstanding visions of women's aging and older age, is, I argue, usefully elucidated via the concept of the "counterfeit." Like "senility," the "counterfeit" slid from the neutral toward the pejorative over the course of the nineteenth century; as Mary McAleer Balkun explains in *The American Counterfeit: Authenticity and Identity in American Literature and Culture*, "Counterfeiting is associated with making and with reproduction. . . . In addition, 'counterfeit' has associations with monetary systems and consumption, with faith, with the theatre, and with art," a distinct set of connotations that distinguish from it from other forms of fraudulence, such as the impostor (which "suggests becoming someone else" in a more exclusively pejorative sense) (7–8). In the machine age processes of industrialization placed matters of authenticity and reproduction at the center of concern (Walter Benjamin's influential essay "The Work of Art in the Age of Mechanical Reproduction" is close at hand here). While certain aspects of counterfeiting have long been criminalized (e.g., the production of unsanctioned currency, a pursuit George Gissing would depict in his

1889 novel *The Nether World*) or the subject of deep intellectual misgivings (e.g., Plato's contempt for mimetic forms and rhetoricians in *The Republic*, a species of disapproval echoed by Leo Tolstoy in his late essay "What is Art?" [1896, English trans. 1900]), its definitions are not exclusively tied to the negative connotations of fakery.[6]

But how is the counterfeit implicated in the matter of human aging and its literary representation? In a series of lively readings of Anglo-American literary texts published between 1880 and 1930, Balkun shows how an obsession with the genuine and its other, the counterfeit, reflects acute anxieties around authenticity as an organizing category for both objects and selfhood. The counterfeit woman, I propose, is the materialization of a new kind of female subject for whom chronological age is somehow at odds with the true self that lies beneath sham appearances, a decoupling made possible by the breakdown of separate spheres of gender and temporality alike. In her most extreme form, the counterfeit woman embodies—or is exposed as embodying—the sham youth at the basis of the aesthetics of senility.

Such conceptualizations are especially evident in a certain genre of satirical literature motivated by the perceived demographic reality of "odd" women at the end of the nineteenth century. Take for example this unsigned "Character Note: The New Woman," published in *Cornhill* in 1894: "She is young, of course. She looks older than she really is. And she calls herself a woman . . . Novissima's chief characteristic is her unbounded satisfaction" (365). The "Character Note" begins by drawing attention to the female body and above all the instability of her apparent age ("older than she really is"). Like Nordau, *Cornhill* forewarns its reader that the treachery of such women begins with their refusal to adhere to the phenotypes of age. Similarly, "The Seven Ages of Woman (As Sir James Crichton Browne Seems Prophetically to See Them)," published in the May 14, 1892 issue of *Punch*, re-imagines Strickland's naïve visualization of woman's life-course using a now-familiar intertextual source:

> Woman's world's a stage,
> And modern women will be ill-cast players;
> They'll have new exits and strange entrances,
> And one She will play many mannish parts,
> And these her Seven Ages. . . .
>   Last scene of all,
> That ends this strange new-fangled history,
> Is sheer unwomanliness, mere sex-negation—
> Sans love, sans charm, sans grace, sans everything.

The poem's subtitle manifests a further inflection of Strickland's and Shakespeare's texts through the recent medical lectures delivered by James Crichton-Browne, a renowned psychiatrist and one of Charles Darwin's most significant correspondents. Crichton-Browne's lecture on "Sex in Education" at the Medical Society of London, published the previous week in *The British Medical Journal* (May 7, 1892), referred to differences in "cerebral physiology" and the female susceptibility to "overpressure" as the reason women ought to be protected from physical exertions and "brain work" (Crichton-Browne, "Sex" 951–952). Nervous degeneration and dementias were the inevitable result of "confus[ed]" new academic policies aimed at accepting women into universities, he argued: "Woe betide the generation that springs from mothers among whom gross nervous degenerations abound!" (953). Crichton-Browne's longstanding professional interest in senile dementias further informs *Punch*'s appropriation of his name in the context of this anti-feminist parody. His lectures on "Mental and Cerebral Diseases" were published in *The British Medical Journal* in 1874 and, along with Bucknill and Tuke's *A Manual of Psychological Medicine* (1858), constituted some of the most extensive considerations of diseases in older age prior to the publication of Charcot's lectures in English several years later. In *The Prevention of Senility* (1905), Crichton-Browne argues that interruptions to fertility and reproduction—iterations of the "mere sex-negation" *Punch* lampoons here—accelerates the onset of pathological aging. "Depend on it," writes Crichton-Browne, "the best anti-septic against senile decay is an active interest in human affairs, and those keep young longest who love most. It is a cogent argument against celibacy and the limitation of families that they deprive old age of those vernal influences in which parents renew their youth" (*Senility* 36).

Punch's parody therefore puns upon both medicalized and dramaturgical prescriptions of women's "ill-cast[ing]." A comparable intertextual logic is employed in this later example, published in *Pick-Me-Up* in April 1897, which lambasts the "needless" extrication of female subjectivity from its traditional temporal moorings:

> Last act of all, a woman *new* but old—
> Old in that all the grace of youth has gone,
> A thing that wears the outer garb of men,
> Yet owneth but man's worsest qualities,
> That preaches doctrines, needless and unclean,
> The which herself but half doth understand,
> She apes all manly sport, disgusting men,

Wears cigarette in mouth, eyeglasses in eye,
Prepares herself a sad unloved old age,
Sans womanhood, sans taste, sans everything. (38, emphasis in
   original)

Taken together, it is clear that the purpose of these parodies is not just to demonstrate "that the New Woman forfeits everything that is attractive," as Patricia Marks argues (12), but also that such women exist in a temporal state that does not actually recognize them as women. *Pick-Me-Up*'s reference to *aping* itself connotes the amplified counterfeiting of such female subjects. "[T]hey that dy maids, must lead Apes in Hell," writes John Donne in *Paradoxes and Problems*, a formulation that was invoked in Shakespeare's comedies (*Much Ado About Nothing*, *The Taming of the Shrew*) and in cultural parlance more generally. Gwendolyn B. Needham notes that the proverb was most likely a seventeenth-century pronatalist adage that condemned celibacy as a "positive evil" or fraudulent ideal (107). As "apes" of the original masculine form, these counterfeit women—like the literary form that ridicules them—present a surfeit of signifiers evacuated of meaning, a spurious imitation of the "real distinguished thing" (to use Henry James's formulation): both the majestically reproductive female body and the masculine subject of Shakespeare's source text.

Of course, the discourse of sham-womanliness has long been a part of misogynist critiques of feminism. A century earlier, Richard Polwhele's *The Unsex'd Females, a Poem* (1798) attacked female public figures like Mary Wollstonecraft, Charlotte Smith, and Anna Letitia Barbauld for their sympathies with the Jacobin movement, while noting with approval the virtues of "proper ladies" whose sense of decorum remained unsullied by distasteful political dalliances (Elizabeth Montagu, Ann Radcliffe, and Fanny Burney among them). Almost exactly one century later, a new tactic is added to this model of literary reactionism. Where Rosalind/Ganymede "counterfeit[s] to be a man" in *As You Like It* (4.3.171) by cross-dressing in costume, the unseemly and subversive subject of these *fin de siècle* parodies further disowns her gendered identity by confusing the aging process as well ("a woman *new* but old"). A catalogue of signs further betrays the abject symbolics of older age. In place of Rosalind's disguising of femininity under male vestments, the New Woman's body functions as a deceitful sheath ("outer garb") that cloaks the true age stamp of the woman under scrutiny. Furthermore, the counterfeit speaks to the idea of multitudes (as opposed to the individual impostor) in a manner consistent with this book's interest in thinking through aging via the apertures opened up by nineteenth-century considerations of population and massified life. Herein lies the essence of senility as a *fin de siècle* aesthetic, and the position occupied by the "Woman Question" within this period's senile topography: by rejecting the compulsory reproductivity associated with the "grace[ful]" state of female youth, an entire class of counterfeit women inhabit their demented future state in the present.

"So old? Or so young? Which?"

Historian of medicine Jesse Ballenger has shown how the late-nineteenth-century medicalization of senility was increasingly understood as a product of civilization. Instead of regarding increased lifespan as a triumph of science and social hygiene, such pathologized apprehensions of aging signaled instead a "narrative of ironic progress" (Ballenger 60). To speak of women's unsuccessful aping at this time therefore draws on multiple discourses of ironic progress, from biological and psychological degeneration to the increasingly misfit iconographic conventions of women's aging. The counterfeit youth I've been describing is one such symptom of the *fin de siècle*'s fixation on the prospect of progress gone awry. In his groundbreaking *Clinical Lectures of Senile and Chronic Diseases* (first published in French, 1867; English trans. 1881), physician Jean-Martin Charcot announced that his aim was to "make clear the *peculiar stamp* which old age impresses on all manifestations of disease," a germane choice of words in the context of establishing the nascent discipline of geriatrics (35, emphasis added).[7] The will to truth implied by Charcot's assertion—how is the human body branded by the passage of time?—expresses the shadow-role played by visions of the counterfeit in *fin de siècle* representations of aging. Like chapter 1's discussion of Godwin's immortal, at the *fin de siècle* female bodies removed from the reproductive circuit—the spinster, the odd woman, and the New Woman—could be similarly understood as subjects who effectively scrambled the reliability of a chronological age stamp.[8]

Take, for example, the conclusion of George Gissing's 1893 novel *The Odd Women*, which describes thirty-three-year-old Rhoda Nunn, the now-resolute celibate and co-founder of a flourishing London typing school for women, holding the infant daughter of another young woman, Monica Madden. As I will discuss shortly, Monica's ill-fated marriage was the partial catalyst for her untimely death and Rhoda has traveled to the countryside to visit Monica's older sisters, now guardians of the orphaned newborn. The novel's final lines read:

Whilst Miss Madden went into the house to prepare hospitalities, Rhoda, still nursing, sat down on a garden bench. She gazed intently at those diminutive features, which were quite placid and relaxing in soft drowsiness. The dark, bright eye was Monica's. And as the baby sank into sleep, Rhoda's vision grew dim; a sigh made her lips quiver, and once more she murmured, "Poor little child!" (332)

The Odd Women concludes with an image that conjures the Christian iconography of the Madonna and child; yet Rhoda's uncharacteristic grief, prompted by the memory of Monica she discerns in the baby's physiognomy, evokes in equal part a grim Pietà. Critics have long discussed the radical ambivalence of the novel's conclusion, debating whether it betrays a message of muted optimism or unconcealed pessimism concerning the "Woman Question." Like the inscrutable "dark, bright" eye Rhoda beholds, this Baby New Year embodies indeterminacy. Gissing deftly refuses final comment on the implications of a future cradled by such brave new ways.

Many twenty-first-century readers will read in Rhoda Nunn an admirable, if problematic, figure of protofeminist emancipation. Yet Rhoda invokes other contortions of meaning as well. On the one hand, this "nursing" figure of maternity reflects the longstanding primacy of women in the context of population theory, be it Montesquieu's procreative matron or (for very different reasons) Malthus's revered spinster. On the other hand, in the *fin de siècle* context I have been describing, the conspicuously named Rhoda Nunn also stands forward as a kind of prematurely, and therefore pathologically, aged woman capable only of holding other people's offspring. Women like Rhoda—the New Woman, odd women, and those like Monica, who betrayed inklings of sympathy toward such alien subjectivities—authorized broader suspicions that unnatural proclivities were effecting the degeneration not just of individuals but of England and Europe more broadly. Rhoda is the embodiment of a compromised, even non-existent future—an inceptive example of how the biopolitics of older age get yoked into debates concerning the approaching horde of new (and New) women. Whereas the childless bachelor Adrian in Mary Shelley's *The Last Man* represented an exemplary Malthusian subject, Monica's infant daughter occupies the arms of a woman with no reproductive future—a state of being that, in the context of the patriarchal temporality that typifies the Victorian period, is equivalent to no future at all. As Grant Allen argued about spinsters in "Plain Words on the Woman Question" (1889), "We ought always clearly to bear in mind—men and women alike—that to all time the vast majority of women must be wives and mothers. . . . [I]f either class must be sacrificed to the other, it is the spinsters whose type perishes with them that should be sacrificed to the matrons who carry on the life and qualities of the species" (456). In the eyes of many at the *fin de siècle*, Rhoda, and to a certain extent, the odd woman-in-waiting she holds, instantiates a populace that announced the end of population itself. As Allen continues: "she is an abnormality, not the woman of the future" (367).

Critics have long appreciated Gissing's fidelity to realist detail, and *The Odd Women*, like his novels *New Grub Street* (1891) and *The Nether World* (1889) before it, testifies to the life of the lower-middle class at the close of the nineteenth century. A 1948 essay on Gissing's oeuvre begins gloomily—"In the shadow of the atomic bomb it is not easy to talk confidently about progress"—but in the wake of the Second World War, with its decades of hostile military and political impasse that have come to pass, George Orwell nevertheless points to Gissing's novels for evidence "that the present age is a good deal better than the last one" (428–429).[9] While not a "masterpiece," Orwell concedes (429), *The Odd Women* presents a startling dramatization of the social conditions responsible for shaping human and especially women's lives at this time: "An elderly spinster crowns a useless life by taking to drink; a pretty young girl marries a man old enough to be her father; a struggling schoolmaster puts off marrying his sweetheart until both of them are middle-aged and withered; . . . in each case the ultimate reason for the disaster lies in obeying the accepted social code, or in not having enough money to circumvent it" (430). Orwell's identification of the connections between money and the social conventions of marriage has influenced many readers' assessment of this novel. Yet I want to draw out how aging, older age, and gender are also at the heart of "the disaster" Orwell explains, because in multiple ways *The Odd Women* invokes age as a means of defining obsolescing models of female subjectivity.

The 1861 census had concluded that there existed at least half a million more women than marriageable men due to factors including emigration and military service (Kranidis 37). A variety of such "superfluous" women constitute the main characters of *The Odd Women*. Upon their father's sudden death at the end of chapter 1, the rural middle-class Madden sisters find themselves completely unprovided for. Without marriage prospects, sufficient education, or practical training, the eldest sisters find themselves seriously struggling to maintain a modest veneer of respectability in London's urban maze. Meanwhile, Monica, the youngest, begins working prolonged hours in a drapery shop among the most desperately sliding lower-middle-class women. An unexpected marriage proposal from Edmund Widdowson, a nervous bachelor twenty-two years her senior, promises to relieve Monica from such drudgery, but another possibility also emerges in the form of training at a typing school run by the iconoclastic feminist Rhoda Nunn. Despite temptations to follow in Rhoda's footsteps, Monica, now pregnant and miserable within the confines of her convenient and utterly conventional marriage to Widdowson, embarks upon a doomed extramarital affair. In a parallel plot, Rhoda is also tempted to combine the demands of women's liberation with matrimony by way of an enticingly egalitarian courtship with Everard, her co-founder Mary Barfoot's outwardly progressive cousin. The demands of love are ultimately incommensurate with Rhoda's feminist principles and the experimental courtship is abandoned. Everard quickly marries a conventionally accomplished young woman, while Rhoda returns to the business of training women for the workplace.

Gissing's novel is conspicuously fixated on the external signs of aging, which, I argue, speaks to its broader concerns with the instability of gender, temporality, and notions of progress catalyzed by the "Woman Question." As is often the case with Gissing, economics binds together these elements of aging and gender. Gissing immediately signals the compromised futurity of the eldest Madden sisters by the hastened encroachment of corporeal senescence. At thirty-five Alice is described as balding and hoarse, while Virginia sits on the precarious threshold of decay: "[s]he was rapidly ageing; her lax lips grew laxer, with emphasis of a characteristic one would rather not have perceived there; her eyes sank into deeper hollows; wrinkles extended their network; the flesh of her neck wore away" (39). If the aging process, like poverty, is most often perceived as a sequence of diminishments, then it is also the insignia of certain immoderations. In Virginia's case, her furtive gin-drinking engenders the jowly superfluity reiterated in Gissing's alliterative upsurge ("lax lips grew laxer"). The signs of older age are most immediately figured as instances of displacement, as features sink, extend, and erode from their earlier forms. Aging is thus a physically transmuted instance of abjection, as parts refuse to remain in their proper place.[10] Such modes of physical attrition run directly counter to ideological decrees like Ruskin's that neatly scaffolded both the bodies and lives of women into separate spheres.

Only thirty-three, Virginia already appears the elderly spinster Orwell describes. Economic hardship exacerbates the transitory assets of youth as poverty, like aging, diminishes the ideal of superabundance that comprised the longstanding female ideal. The elder sisters' monetary and material prudence effectively compensates for, by guarding against, the wasting process of physical aging. Determined to live off only the interest of their humble inheritance (800 pounds), Alice and Virginia's existence comes at the expense of bodily health; the sisters dine on meager rations of boiled potato and conceal their poverty under the pretext of vegetarianism. In one of the novel's most demoralizing scenes, in the cramped space of their shared garret the sisters endeavor to cheer each other by swearing to defend themselves from total degradation:

> "Whatever happens, my dear," said Alice presently, with all the impressiveness of tone she could command, "we must never entrench upon our capital—never—never!"
> "Oh, never! If we grow old and useless—"
> "If no one will give us even board and lodging for our services—"
> "If we haven't a friend to look to," Alice threw in, as though they were answering each other in a doleful litany, "then indeed we shall be glad that nothing tempted us to entrench on our capital! It would just keep us"—her voice sank—"from the workhouse." (44)

Gissing's portrait of these oldening odd women draws a clear connection between economic stability and the aging process. As the abstracted capital of youth diminishes, Alice and Virginia are left with only their economic bolus; as their helplessly practiced refrain insinuates, little difference exists between the impoverished woman and the aged one. Keeping their small financial assets intact is their only hope of staving off the symbolic death that Shakespeare once attributed to "unaccommodated man" (*King Lear* 3.4.99)—a hostile condition of wretchedness perhaps even more likely encountered in the struggle for urban existence at the *fin de siècle* than in the state of external nature. Like *New Grub Street*, where the hourly peal of the workhouse bell is the grim accompaniment to Edwin Reardon's struggle to scrape together a living as a novelist, the specter of the institution threatens a probable future for this new species of women artificially oldened by social inequities as much as the passage of time.

Alice's tactical tenor in this passage is an ironic adaptation of women's capacity to "rule" (as Ruskin would have it) and, more gravely, an indication of the feeble reality of such a gendered marital order against the battle of Victorian life itself. Not incidentally, variations on the word "struggle" appear twenty-three times throughout the novel, an anchoring motif reflective of the social, biological, affective, and economic ideations of battle that *The Odd Women* unblinkingly recounts. Such language also points up the naturalization of the Darwinian "struggle for existence" as a social ideal capable of effacing the misery envisioned in the Malthusian population principle. With few exceptions, in Gissing's novel and beyond, the future possibilities for odd women like Alice and Virginia were not expansive (as promised by budding investments and expanding networks) or even static (as in un-"entrenched" capital), but entirely exhaustive and abjecting ("old and useless").

Twenty-one-year-old Monica reads these grim signs with pitiable erudition. "She thought of her sisters. Their loneliness was for life, poor things. Already they were old; and they would grow older, sadder, perpetually struggling to supplement that dividend from the precious capital—and merely that they might keep alive" (58). Monica's lament highlights the ambiguity of the "dividend" so valuable to her older sisters, as their small allowance only allows them to effectively accumulate a paradoxical stock of diminishing corporeal and affective returns. The sisters are living proof of the naïve fallacy at the heart of organicist visions of progress and growth, strongly associated with midcentury Victorianism and its novelistic productions (as I described in chapter 3). For Alice and Virginia, the accumulation of time is a hopelessly accelerated dissipation. Monica's sense of this diminishment occurs on multiple registers, sympathizing as she does with the social and financial deprivations of these "poor things." However, her own dread contaminates this compassion with an unseemly sort of insight. "Oh!—her heart ached at the misery of such a prospect. How much better if the poor girls had never been born" (58). Monica's morbid hope for her own siblings illustrates a Malthusian position in caricature, aiming to prevent misery not by alleviating conditions of poverty in the present but by curtailing impoverished futures in the womb. Such attitudes obviously held traction at the end of the nineteenth century. Thomas Hardy articulates exactly these ideas in *Jude the Obscure*: consider the elderly aunt who taunts the young Jude with similar notions of the utility and futility of inconvenient lives. "It would ha' been a blessing if Goddy-mighty had took thee too, wi' thy mother and father, poor useless boy!" (Hardy 49). Two years in advance of the austere calculations made by Jude's son, Little Father Time, Gissing's novel voices a kindred recognition of the relationship between poverty, aging, and gender.

Monica sees in the life of her spinster sisters, now multiply subjected to the deformation of numbers, an unconvincing counterfeit of what

Victorian life seemed to promise (her own future was to be otherwise, as her father's sighs pledged to her at five years old: "ah, little Monica! She would be the beauty of the family" [34]). Although more than a decade younger than Alice and Virginia, Monica nevertheless apprehends them as "girls"—fooled, perhaps, by their false optimism (be it the product of Alice's religious devotion or Virginia's alcoholism, which remains a secret until the novel's end). For Monica, the dividend of such a life is the confusion of abject old age ("already they were old; and they would grow older") and nominal childhood ("poor girls"), a condemnation of the historical age and ideological climate that would have her sisters occupy both disenfranchised states at once.

Monica's age appraisal speaks to a concern that underpins *The Odd Women*, namely, the intersection of gender and the reproductive future marriage implies. The generational contrast drawn by the Madden daughters and their mother indicates that the relationship between these coordinates is shifting rapidly. With a wink to the fecund matron that so appalled Malthus, the first chapter ("The Fold and the Shepherd") opens with an indistinct portrait of the abundant Mrs. Madden, late mother to six daughters and devoted wife of Clevedon's country doctor. Gissing immediately evokes, only to eradicate, the life of this "sweet, calm, unpretending woman," of whom the reader only knows that she evokes from husband and daughter a Ruskinian "sigh" of remembrance (31). Then, one crucial detail: "[s]he had known but little repose, and secret anxieties told upon her countenance long before the final collapse of health" (31–32). Gissing never elaborates on the nature of Mrs. Madden's "anxieties" before disappearing her from the narrative altogether: perhaps she suffered the physical toll of birthing and raising several children, or presaged her six daughters' imminent hardships—of Gertrude, Martha, and Isabel readers learn at the outset of chapter 2 that they have died by early adulthood of consumption, a boating accident, and suicide by drowning, respectively—or took it upon herself to assuage her own "sordid cares" with alcohol, as Virginia would. (Gissing imposes a similarly sudden invisibilizing of Marian Yule in the final chapters of *New Grub Street*, thus implying the intention of such narrative silence.)

Not unlike Dr. Madden's "faithful old roadster," the elderly horse whose collapse kills his procrastinating owner and initiates the novel's action, the reader is assured that Mrs. Madden "had fulfilled her function in this wonderful world" through her prolific childbearing. In dying, she achieves the perfect stasis that Ruskin's portrait of femininity aims to capture (31). As Claudia Nelson argues, only the grave "can be the site of a genuinely happy marriage to an arrested child-woman" (74); as a point of contrast, consider Miss Havisham in Dickens's *Great Expectations* who, by not occupying the authorized offstage spaces of matrimony or death, becomes in her old age a grotesque parody of the child-woman.) Beginning with the foisting offstage of Mrs. Madden, *The Odd Women* depends on the specter of Victorian motherhood—the old womanly woman—as an archetype against which to define the contours of a new generation.

Monica's appraisal of her sisters's aged appearance is repeated almost immediately in her first meeting with Edmund Widdowson, but to very different result. A sideways glance reveals him to be "an oldish man, with grizzled whiskers and rather a stern visage" (59), which Monica greets with a fatigued "sigh" (59). His exceptionally polite conversation prompts a return to her physiognomic reading: "How old might he be? After all, he was probably not fifty—perchance not much more than forty" (59). Monica's self-assured evaluation of her sisters' premature decrepitude gives way to an explicit, yet vague, quantitative strategy to gauge the propriety of her unchaperoned public encounter with Widdowson. Their next meeting follows a similar pattern: "Speculating again about his age, Monica concluded that he must be two or three and forty, in spite of the fact that his grizzled beard argued for a higher figure. He had brown hair untouched by any sign of advanced life, his teeth were white and regular, and something—she could not make clear to her mind exactly what—convinced her that he had a right to judge himself comparatively young" (66). The economic dimensions of Monica's calculations are unmistakable. The semi-legibility of Widdowson's age are hitched to his likely class and character, and Monica "speculat[es]" that ultimately the man before her is deserving of the most sympathetic "figure." In both cases, numbers generate for Monica a persuasive narrative of either the comic or tragic sort.

In an 1893 review of *The Odd Women,* Clementina Black writes, "[t]he apparent surplus of women is largely due to the fact that they live longer. If a hundred men and a hundred women were to be born ever[y] year, and if all the men lived to fifty, while all the women lived to fifty-one, there would be a permanent surplus of a hundred women, and yet every one of these might have been married to one of the hundred men born in the same year as herself" (155). In multiple ways, then, life *expectancy* is at the root of the "odd women" debate—be it length of life or the convenient fictions of life's progress in Victorian Britain. Gissing's novel begins with a portrait of the folly of this confusion. Dr. Madden's plan to purchase a life insurance plan "to-morrow" is based upon his assumption that, "at the age of forty-nine . . . [m]ight he not reasonably count on ten or fifteen more years of activity?" (31). This assumption of positive, progressive futurity nevertheless rests on a kind of endless afternoon of the present, a ceaselessly active growth that justifies the ignorant deferral of the future: "Human beings are not destined to struggle for ever like beasts of prey. Give them time; let civilization grow" (32). The irony of Dr. Madden's reassuring words builds with his reading of Tennyson's "The Lotos-Eaters" in a voice, Gissing notes, that "blended with the song of a thrush"—an ominous signal to any reader with an ear to Hardy's "The Darkling Thrush," his elegiac landscape poem on the termination of the nineteenth century (35). The growth of civilization that Dr. Madden does not survive another week to see is a future almost wholly unable to accommodate "redundant" women.

In Gissing's London, where demography and social inequities united to both olden and impoverish a growing number of *fin de siècle* women, Eliot's pastoral view of re-pairing seems a distant, unworkable ideal. Where young and old, or new and old, might have once been joined, in terms of the implied and optimistic futurity implied by the narrative of development "youth" was, for a growing number of young women, an unobtainable state of life. Yet *The Odd Women* also demonstrates the folly of quantitative strategies that would reduce individuals to the implied narrative of numbers. Gissing stages this tactic most overtly upon introducing Rhoda Nunn. "Younger only by a year or two than Virginia, she was yet far from presenting any sorrowful image of a person on the way to old-maidenhood. She had a clear though pale skin, a vigorous frame, a brisk movement—all the signs of fairly good health. Whether or not she could be called a comely woman might have furnished matter for male discussion; the prevailing voice of her own sex would have denied her charm of feature" (Gissing 48). As Gissing's mention of "male discussion" expresses, both Dr. Madden's imprudent hopefulness and Monica's relentless cynicism contrast starkly with Rhoda Nunn's (dis) engagement with numbers of both the individual and population-based sort. Rhoda speaks both frankly and vaguely of her own age, and in so doing indicates the way such enumerations serve to limit women's agency. "So it is your birthday?" she remarks, upon first meeting Monica. "I no longer keep count of mine, and couldn't tell you without a calculation what I am exactly. It doesn't matter, you see. Thirty-one or fifty-one is much the same for a woman who has made up her mind to live alone and work steadily for a definite object" (63). Rhoda dismisses the acute age appraisal by which Monica calculates her sisters' curtailed future, by turning on herself the generously obfuscating gaze that Monica had permitted Widdowson during their encounter. (There is, of course, considerable irony in Rhoda's pronouncement: she is indeed thirty-one, and perfectly cognizant of her own age, but she also occupies the perspective held by other men in the novel like Widdowson and Bevis who insist upon regarding Monica and her sisters through the disenfranchising Ruskinian gaze of girlhood.) Against the symbolic oldening and social death that threaten to eclipse Virginia and Alice, work—not the drudgery Monica fears, but real, useful, self-actualizing work—counteracts the incapacitating onset of figurative and perhaps even physiological aging.

By explicitly linking age with the capacity to make a living, Rhoda sidesteps the discursive life-staging that structures individual women's life around courtship, matrimony, and motherhood, and would discard those faulty specimens that find themselves unpaired in the process. Such a revised outlook is evident in Rhoda's calculatedly shocking comments on the hard conditions for this class of women:

> "I wish girls fell down and died of hunger in the streets, instead of creeping to their garrets and the hospitals. I should like to see their dead bodies collected together in some open place for the crowd to stare at."
>
> Monica gazed at her with wide eyes.
>
> "You mean, I suppose, that people would try to reform things."
>
> "Who knows? Perhaps they might only congratulate each other that a few of the superfluous females had been struck off.—Do they give you any summer holiday?" (62)

Monica imagines that Rhoda's modest proposal is intended to solicit some civic strategy for repairing wasted female life, but Rhoda's view of the "surplus"—be it the superfluous quantifying of age or of population more generally—refuses to repeat Dr. Madden's error of imagining reform as a predestined or even probable inevitability. Rhoda's casual redirection of the conversation toward Monica's working conditions at the drapery shop emphasizes her ironic take on the value of increasing the visibility of an abject class, a strategy of rebellion just as prone to fortifying collective aversion toward women's lot as provoking meaningful societal change. This conversational strategy is suggestive of Gissing's own skepticism concerning the effectiveness of literature and specifically realism as a method of effecting social reform. In an essay written two years after *The Odd Women* was published Gissing states, "Public opinion no longer constrains a novelist to be false to himself. . . . [I]t is purely a matter for his private decision whether he will write as the old law dictates or show life its image as he beholds it" ("Realism," 316). The indefinite outcome of literary writing and its interpretation results in a style that for Gissing "is simultaneously personal and mediated," as Susan E. Cook has argued (458). Rhoda, who is to some extent Gissing's avatar throughout *The Odd Women*, adopts this role by embodying the "rhetoric of apparent paradox" required to realize realism's sincere and productive indeterminacy (Matz 100).

Rather than viewing this growing class of counterfeit women in the hopelessly dismissive terms of redundancy, Rhoda imagines for them a vital social role. "So many *odd* women—no making a pair with them. The pessimists call them useless, lost, futile lives. I, naturally—being one of them myself—take another view. I look upon them as a great reserve. When one woman vanishes in matrimony, the reserve offers a substitute for the world's work. True, they are not all trained yet—far from it. I want to help in that—to train the reserve" (64, emphasis in original). In contrast to Monica's stigmatization of the typing school as "an old-maid factory" (75), Rhoda's strategy of massification takes on a revolutionary tenor very different from the cultural death drive Monica invokes, or the then-ubiquitous interpretation of surplus women as a "burden" on the state (Kranidis 37). Rhoda's appeal to the "reserve" refashions the obsolescent language of women's temporal sphere in terms of economic potential, rather than as embodiments of cultural decline. Where Monica fears the typing school because it produces non-marriageable and thus counterfeit women, Rhoda's view is that her work provides the means of infusing the social sphere with a new class of legitimate workers. Significantly, she gestures to Monica's reluctant contemplation of the school's two Remington machines by backtracking on her feminist stridency, indulging Monica's sense of matrimonial eligibility by referring to the latter's birthday: "But you are still a young girl, Monica. My best wishes!" (63).

Rhoda's age indeterminacy is emphasized yet again in the context of her relationship with Miss Mary Barfoot, her friend and co-founder of the typing school. Ten years older than Rhoda, Mary Barfoot has a devotion to improving women's lot no less steadfast than her younger counterpart's. Unlike Rhoda, however, Mary accepts marriage as a continuing necessity ("My dear, after all we don't desire the end of the race" [76], an argument with which Rhoda unpersuasively concurs). Such differences indicate the generational partitioning that distinguishes Rhoda's feminism from the moderate pragmatism of her partner. "Oh, I am a very old-fashioned woman," Mary says, "Women have thought as I do at any time in history. Miss Nunn has much more zeal for womanhood militant" (106). These discrepancies are conspicuous in their differing reactions to the failed romantic affair of a lapsed former student, which results in the student's eventual suicide. Whereas Rhoda views the woman's death as a necessary judgment (what else could such a foolish reader of romantic novels have expected, abandoning the only mode of life that promised her an economically independent future?), Mary grieves deeply and is alarmed by her companion's "severe logic" (147). "Miss Barfoot smiled sadly. 'How young you are! Oh, there is far more than ten years between our ages, Rhoda! In spirit you are a young girl, and I an old woman. No, no; we will not quarrel. Your companionship is far too precious to me, and I dare to think that mine is not without value for you'" (151).

Where Alice and Virginia are struck by Rhoda's masculine style ("The most wonderful person! She is quite like a *man* in energy and resources. I never imagined that one of our sex could resolve and plan and act as she does!" [57]), Mary eschews such Ruskinian tendencies and views Rhoda's ideological comportment through the temporal lens of age. Rhoda's indeterminant age stamp speaks not only to her subversion of traditional gender roles, but her invasion of the temporal (and at times affective) sphere typically and more comfortably associated with the masculine. In certain respects Rhoda most closely resembles Mary's cousin, Everard, whose modern orientation is reflected in a similar constellation of indeterminacy. Both enjoy considerable freedom of mobility (Everard travels internationally, while Rhoda takes her annual ten-day holiday around England), rejecting the rigid ideological demands of life-staging. Everard, however, enjoys further privileges bestowed by his masculinity that safeguard from scrutiny his bachelor status. Only one or two years older than Rhoda, Everard has yet to enter the prime of his life (whereas the elder Madden sisters, his age-peers, are effectively in their twilight years). The different stakes associated with male and female age are apparent upon his return to England, when Mary gently inquires into the "social usefulness" of his anticipated plans:

> "What are you going to do?" she asked of him good-naturedly.
> "To do? You mean, how do I propose to employ myself? I have nothing whatever in view, beyond enjoying life."
> "At your age?"
> "So young? Or so old? Which?"

> "So young, of course. You deliberately intend to waste your life?"
>
> "To enjoy it, I said. I am not prompted to any business or profession; that's all over for me; I have learnt all I care to of the active world." (104)

Like Tennyson's lotus-eaters, Everard repudiates any sense of futurity's mandatory contours, claiming the right to "an infinite series of modes of living. A ceaseless exercise of all one's faculties of pleasure" (104). The scrambled hermeneutics of age further recalls the senile degenerate life that so disturbed Nordau; Mary's uncertainty as to whether such retirement is the consequence of youthful heedlessness or aged exhaustion reveals a confusion of age-states that eventually links Everard's character with more the fantastical endowments of a Dorian Gray or St. Leon. Unlike the troubling age-stamp of several female characters in *The Odd Women*, Everard's apparent age only prompts a mild, passing concern as to its implied future narrative. A life that can be indistinguishably wasted or enjoyed is one in which time's passing is simply a temporary reprieve: a luxurious state of perpetuity denied to women both within and beyond the marriage market.

Everard's counterfeit pursuit of Rhoda ("just to prove her [feminist] sincerity" [115]) indicates how deeply the matter of human temporality is convolved in the matter of marriage in the British novel. Each of the three marriage plots represented in the novel is conspicuously marked by matters of age. Widdowson's hopes that his "little girl" will uphold the Ruskinian values dogmatically espoused by the "old bear" (171) collapse upon Monica's growing determination to lead a moderately independent life. Monica's marriage to her "elderly admirer" testifies to the disastrous inequities of the woman-child and the two-decades-older mature man—a disparity further coded in literary terms (he reads Walter Scott, she reads Ouida) (171). The Mickelthwaites, by contrast, present by far the happiest portrait of matrimony, as reflected in the alignment of Mick and Fanny's probable futures. Prevented from marrying in their youth due to poverty, the two forty-year-olds conclude their seventeen-year engagement with a painfully modest wedding ceremony wholly divergent in tone from the Widdowsons' bleak nuptials. Everard's former mathematics teacher is elated: "I am renewing my youth. Nay, for the first time I am youthful. I never had time for it before. At the age of sixteen I began to teach in a school, and ever since I have pegged away at it, school and private. Now luck has come to me, and I feel five-and-twenty. When I was really five-and-twenty,

I felt forty" (112). Mick's autobiography begins in a state of counterfeit youth, a case of oldening imposed by the wasting consequence of poverty. The decent pecuniary success of his mathematics textbook illustrates how the expenditures of labor may also be converted into the symbolics of youth and its figurative capital, an arithmetic at the heart of his calculations regarding his own real versus chronological age. Mick's "luck" transforms the wasting grind of teaching into the enjoyable labor of education, a transformation that coincides with the Malthusian ideal of entering into marriage at the time not of peak reproductive status but of stable financial assets and prospects instead.

His rejuvenation comes well in advance of his fiancée Fanny's, however, as Everard's observant eye is quick to notice. "At three-and-twenty she had possessed a sweet, simple comeliness on which any man's eye would have rested with pleasure; at forty she was wrinkled, hollow-cheeked, sallow, indelible weariness stamped upon her brow and lips. She looked much older than Mary Barfoot, though they were just of an age. And all this for want of a little money" (142). In contrast to Everard's watchfulness—pitying, on the one hand, but also suspiciously gazing on the other—Mick's adoration elevates his bride in a way that only serves to affirm their temporal mutuality. "Oh, Fanny! But I have never thought of Fanny as a separate person. Upon my word, now I think of it, I never have. Fanny and I have been one for ages" (142). Mick's formulation invokes Aristophanes's fable (discussed in chapter 3) by binding together the simultaneity of personal histories and chronological age. Like Mick's, Fanny's age stamp is softened to a near-Ruskinian condition by the time Everard returns to visit the happy couple a few months later. "Mrs. Micklethwaite was no longer so distressingly old; an expression that resembled girlish pleasure lit up her countenance as she stepped forward; nay, if he mistook not, there came a gentle warmth to her cheek, and the momentary downward glance was as graceful and modest as in a youthful bride. Never had Barfoot approached a woman with more finished courtesy, the sincere expression of his feeling" (188). Like Monica's, Everard's observations indicate his own falling back on traditional visions of youthful women's beauty (Gissing's own habits of irony are at work in this passage, if readers mistake not). Yet Everard's typically ironic stance drops for a moment, struck by the older couple's happy mutuality. Once again, their perfect compatibility is coded by reference to reading material. Speaking of Mick's plans to write a series of mathematical textbooks, the couple joke over their love of numbers: "We will gossip about sines and co-sines before we die" (143).

Individual happiness and apparent youthening aside, however, whether the Micklethwaites' "Malthusian marriage" (Niles, "Malthusian" 295) should be taken as a model remains unclear. *The Odd Women* remains silent on the ramifications of this resolution to women's redundancy. As the Micklethwaites demonstrate, marriage in older age interrupts, scrambles, or even (and I am aware of my anachronism here) queers the ideological age-based expectations traditionally associated both with the institution of marriage itself, which insists on the compulsory misalignment of male and female temporalities required for reproduction.

For these reasons, I propose, Gissing stages the third "marriage" plot involving Everard and Rhoda, who are very close in age and at least superficially interested in the possibility of a progressive union unencumbered by the drag of traditional arrangements: "the old story," as Everard twice describes it (206, 273), the "old, idle form" (272), with its "old word[s]" (190), a provocative echo of Gissing's own impatience with the "old law" of realism mentioned earlier.[11] Through Everard Gissing paints a wizened portrait of the matrimonial institution; Rhoda is not fully convinced that new customs would be any more compatible with a model of progress that disqualifies traditional visions of female temporality. "Love of husband—perhaps of child. There must be more than that," Rhoda says as she contemplates the futurity promised by marriage (271). The reproductive circuit enabled by matrimony gives birth only to old and sterile ideas—a counterfeit kind of progress indeed.

The "battle" (277) that materializes between Rhoda and Everard is less a troubled courtship than a struggle for the rights to non-reproductive mechanisms of progress. An engineer by training, Everard disparages Rhoda's conflation of personal and professional futures by implying the sham emancipation that typing represents:

> "What is your work? Copying with a type-machine, and teaching others to do the same—isn't that it?"
>
> "The work by which I earn money, yes. But if it were no more than that—"
>
> "Explain, then."
>
> Passion was overmastering him as he watched the fine scorn in her eyes. He raised her hand to his lips.
>
> "No!" Rhoda exclaimed with sudden wrath. "Your respect—oh, I appreciate your respect!" (195–196)

Like the ambiguous hermeneutics of alchemy (which mapped the immortal St. Leon's sterile future a century earlier), at the *fin de siècle* the typewriter stands forward as a mechanism of counterfeit progress: on the one hand, marking women's advancement into new temporal and spatial realms and, on the other, the animating engine of the old-maid factory once envisioned by Monica. Rhoda's refusal to reduce her "work" (itself a forked word in the history of women's industry, from the eighteenth-century domestic occupation of needlework to the new problematics of "labour" that typewriting connotes), to either the barren alternatives of capitalistic or matrimonial gain, generates an impasse that culminates in her refusal of his marriage offer. "We should only play at defying it," Rhoda concludes; like Everard, she is unable to respect what they behold as counterfeit advancement (271). The wedding ring and the typewriter, like the bioeconomics of women's labor they imply, are obligatory, productive, but ultimately untransformative vectors of social progress.

This impasse is most wretchedly represented by Monica's dismal prospects at the end of the novel. Pregnant, trapped in a stultifying marriage, and now a humiliated failure of a mistress, the youngest Madden sister is awakened to a series of realizations. The fiasco imposes a kind of existential senescence that her chronological youth weirdly belies. In her final conversation with Rhoda, Monica "hope[s]" rather than fears that she is dying: "I can see nothing before me. I don't wish to live" (314). The financial poverty that threatens other oldened characters in Gissing's novel is transmuted into the impoverished prospects of matrimonial culture. This particular refusal of the future—her own, and the one implicit in her ensuing oath that "I shall not love my child"—perverts the temporal expectations of the nexus of hope, youth, and progress (315). Two years later, Hardy's *Jude the Obscure* would portray an analogous negation. As Jude recollects the physician's words in the aftermath of Little Father Time's notorious murder-suicide, "The doctor says there are such boys springing up among us—boys of a sort unknown in the last generation—the outcome of new views of life. They seem to see all its terrors before they are old enough to have staying power to resist them. He says it is the beginning of the coming universal wish not to live" (Hardy 365). In the *fin de siècle* landscape, there exist a new species of little boys, and little girl-women, for whom the exhausted impoverishment of traditional institutions inscribes their corruption of the future in the lineaments of a new, counterfeit youth. The collapse of such traditional vehicles of cultural progress—be it marriage, reproduction, technology, even literary realism—is evinced in such obscene forms of abject senility.

The Coming of Age

In a stirring speech to her students, Mary Barfoot links women's active participation in the world with an overtly temporalized subject. "The old types of womanly perfection are no longer helpful to us," she rallies (152). "There must be a new type of woman, active in every sphere of life: a new worker out in the world, a new ruler of the home. Of the old ideal virtues we can retain many, but we have to add to them those which have been thought appropriate only in men. . . . Let the responsibility for disorder rest on those who have made us despise our old selves" (153). Entitled "Woman as an Invader," Mary's speech articulates how the erosion of separate spheres demands a transformation that prepares women not only for rule but also for battle—an invasion of the temporal as well as social spheres of gender. Her speech is, of course, a testament to the *fin de siècle* hopes for the New Woman, yet Gissing's novel quietly hints at literature's role in the realization of such progress, be it counterfeit or otherwise. Does literature serve as an agent of change—does it enable its ideas, subjects, and methods of representation to grow, age, perish—or does it simply embalm the status quo? *The Odd Women*, like other literary texts of this time, relies on the language of war, conflict, and struggle to reflect upon the ways in which progress, specifically as it is figured through age, becomes legible to the literary imagination. From parodies of women new but old to Gissing's unblinking realism, literary writing helped articulate a fierce struggle between ideations of the past and future that often materialized in terms of human aging.

In its emphasis on military imagery—not only in the content of Mary's and Rhoda's speeches, but as evinced in a number of the novel's chapter titles ("A Camp of the Reserve," "Discord of Leaders," "The Triumph," "A Reinforcement," "Towards the Decisive," "In Ambush," "Retreat With Honour")—*The Odd Women* launches its critique of literature's ability to negotiate relations between the old and new. The specter of Ruskin, as I've discussed, haunts the male and female characters of *The Odd Women* alike, yet other intertexts are also at stake in this novel concerning the course of progress. Tennyson's "The Lotos-Eaters" provides a crucial indicator of the misguided placidity by which Dr. Madden recounts his own life expectancy and that he presumes for his own daughters. Yet other Tennysonian visions hover in the margins as well. If "The Burden of Futile Souls" (the title of chapter 28) points directly to the ostensibly "useless, lost, futile" lives of Britain's odd women, Rhoda's wish to confront gawking onlookers with heaps of dead women echoes Tennyson's own narrative of futility portrayed in his 1854 poem, "The Charge of the Light Brigade."[12] His indictment of the disastrously administrated Crimean war concluded with a tribute to the ageless courage of the doomed "six hundred" killed at the Battle of Balaclava just six weeks earlier:

> When can their glory fade?
> O the wild charge they made!
> All the world wonder'd.
> Honour the charge they made!
> Honour the Light Brigade,
> Noble six hundred! (50–55)

The implied alignment of superfluous soldiers and women builds with the fact that in Gissing's novel, Rhoda's residence is located directly across the street from Chelsea Hospital, an institution dedicated to the care of elderly British soldiers since its founding in 1682 (a location Gissing mentions twice in his meticulously mapped novel of London). However, Tennyson's consecration of those wasted soldiers lies far from Rhoda's trenchant irony. In fact, Rhoda's realist fondness for her own "ragged regiment" (Gissing 76) has much more in common with a rarely cited rejoinder to Tennyson's poem. Almost forty years after "The Charge of the Light Brigade" was published, and three years before Gissing's *The Odd Women*, Rudyard Kipling's "The Last of the Light Brigade" (1890) reads as a sobering remedy to Tennyson's soaring romance of literary immortality. In Kipling's rendering, the "tattered and frayed" remains of the Light Brigade (line 19), now aged, destitute, and infirm, return to entreat "the Master-singer" (14) to now write of their dire poverty and neglect:

> The old Troop-Sergeant was spokesman, and "Beggin' your
>   pardon," he said,
> "You wrote o' the Light Brigade, sir. Here's all that isn't dead.
> An' it's all come true what you wrote, sir, regardin' the mouth
>   of hell;
> For we're all of us nigh to the workhouse, an' we thought
>   we'd call an' tell.
>
> "No, thank you, we don't want food, sir; but couldn't you
>   take an' write

> A sort of 'to be continued' and 'see next page' o' the fight?
> We think that someone has blundered, an' couldn't you tell
>   'em how?
> You wrote we were heroes once, sir. Please, write we are starving now."
> (Kipling, "The Last of the Light Brigade" 21–28)

Kipling's riposte undercuts Tennyson's gallant elevation of the Light Brigade, underscoring how the original poem's epic mode makes it impossible to account for the embodied, corporeal reality of aging. Like Ruskin's ageless, impotent angel-woman, Tennyson's six-hundred-odd soldiers remain locked in a state of majestic youth unable to admit time's diminutions ("They felt that life was fleeting; they knew not that art was long, / That though they were dying of famine, they lived in deathless song" [Kipling, 5–6]). In contrast to Strickland's effacement of female mortality by means of her reverent pastiche in "The Seven Ages of Woman," Kipling's depiction of the "poor little army" (29) requests a narrative of futurity that confronts the destabilized ideals of both the body and the narrative of progress: in other words, a new textual production literate to the extraliterary human endgame of aging.

Kipling's "The Last of the Light Brigade" reads as an abysmal exemplar of the counterfeit youth of the British literary tradition itself: a travesty of literary grandeur that afflicts not only Tennyson's poetic subject but also his "babbl[ing]," "lisping" readers:

> O thirty million English that babble of England's might,
> Behold there are twenty heroes who lack their food to-night;
> Our children's children are lisping to "honour the charge they
>   made—"
> And we leave to the streets and the workhouse the charge of
>   the Light Brigade! (43–46)

Unlike the "anxiety of influence" Harold Bloom has described, Kipling's response demands not so much a castration of Tennyson's legacy as a textual coda ("to be continued") that acknowledges the literary afterlife of the "The Charge of the Light Brigade" and the fate of its human referents. Kipling returns to Tennyson in the guise of the aged soldiers, with tactics resembling Mary Barfoot's: not calling for revolution, nor a total rejection of the naïve ideals of agelessness, but demanding acknowledgment of lived temporalities that exist beyond the pale of the dominant ideologies that would marginalize them. In Gissing's *The Odd Women,* as Rhoda prepares to take her annual seaside holiday, she exclaims, "I shall doze there for a fortnight, and forget all about the 'so-called nineteenth century'" (121), phrasing that attests to her profound skepticism concerning the progressive maturity of Victorian culture so apparent to conservatives like Greg, Allen, and their ilk.[13] Kipling's "The Last of the Light Brigade" voices a similarly incredulous account of the century's claims to achievement by viewing the discomfiting reproductive juggernaut of generations ("Our children's children") in tandem with the counterfeit, "so-called" progress of a culture that would deny worldly realities obscured by its exalted literary tradition. At the *fin de siècle,* the return of the abjected subject of age—be it in the form of innovatively oldened characters, recrudescent literary forms, or intertextual visitations—is therefore at the heart of both sympathetic and critical representations of the aesthetics of senescence, and its subsequent critical revisioning of literary immortality.

Senile Reading

Kipling's poem, like Gissing's novel, presents a moving homage to the bioeconomical fate of lives that older age fashions into surplus, then burdensome, cohorts. In each, senescence flags the multiple diminishments faced by the degraded classes in the late days of the Victorian period: diminishments that often involved an unseemly silencing, interruption, reversal, quickening, or distortion of the conventional narrative qualities of individual life-course. *The Odd Women* therefore occupies an important position in the nineteenth-century literary history of aging. For an entire class of such persons, Gissing's novel makes clear, the repair of such a demographic and cultural rift may well take the form of a new and paradoxically unreproductive future. Whether art is up to the task of mending this fissured state finds its answer only in Gissing's final, inconclusive image of Rhoda holding Monica's orphan child. Almost three decades before Freud would articulate his theory of the "death drive" in *Beyond the Pleasure Principle* (1920), late-nineteenth-century literature, the novel especially, probed the forked nature of progress by engaging the symbolics and representational tactics of age.

In addition to the naturalistic and parodic texts I have discussed, it is important to recognize the workings of counterfeit youth in other literary modes of this period. George Bernard Shaw's problem play *Mrs. Warren's*

Profession (1893), for instance, investigates the economic reasons underlying the intergenerational conflict between Kitty, a former prostitute and now brothel owner, and her adult daughter Vivie, a recent university graduate returned from studies (exactly the pre-senile demographic that so worried James Crichton-Browne). Shaw's portrait of Vivie's mannish demeanor and Cambridge education denote not only maturity beyond her twenty-two years, but also a weird species of generational misalignment. In the first act, Praed (whom Shaw's stage directions describe as "hardly past middle age" [87]) remarks to Mrs. Warren ("between 40 and 50 . . . an old blackguard of a woman" [95]) and the fifty-year-old Crofts, "I think, you know—if you don't mind my saying so—that we had better get out of the habit of thinking of her as a little girl. You see she has really distinguished herself; and I'm not sure, from what I have seen of her, that she is not older than any of us" (96–97). Praed's reluctance to employ the conventional language of girlhood with reference to Vivie is compounded by his sense of her hypermaturescence, a state of incongruity between self and age generated by her education and, it is fair to assume, by her refusal of two marriage proposals over the course of the play's action (Vivie later describes herself as "permanently unromantic" [149]). Mrs. Warren's amusement at Praed's intimation ("Older than any of us! Well, she has been stuffing you nicely with her importance" [97]) articulates an alternative interpretation: that Vivie's maturity is only a flimsy front for the naïve conviction that life without sex is possible. Of course, these two women (new but old, mother and daughter alike) transgress the heteroreproductive dictates of futurity—Kitty's successful chain of brothels are the material possibility for Vivie's solitary study of mathematics. Neither, however, is prepared to accept the vision of so-called progress the other embodies. The play concludes by emphasizing their solitary futures, quickened by Kitty's desperate plea: "Who is to care for me when I'm old?" (150)

Such counterfeit women, a class whose compulsory oldening compounds their abject non-reproductivity, are doubly counterfeited in the gothic mode, a literary category that vividly registered deep fears concerning the fate of species coded by women's blurring of temporally based identities. In his essay "The Gothic Ghost of the Counterfeit and the Progress of Abjection," Jerrold E. Hogle describes how the counterfeit constitutes the basis of gothic fiction and is "bound up with the ways that *fin de siècle* selves and 'realities' are hollowed out and reconstituted by representations of representations" (497). This "recounterfeiting" or "ghosting" of the counterfeit "virtually *demands* that there be some abjection, since the process of recounterfeiting is always trying to reach beyond its own anomalous situation, its being pulled backwards and forwards, by reusing the very past counterfeits that it keeps rejecting as empty and dead" (505, emphasis in original). This process is evidently at stake in gothicized recapitulations of counterfeit youth, especially those motivated by intense middle-class anxieties involving a new class of unreproductive female subjects.

H. Rider Haggard's imperial fantasy *She* (1886–7), for example, provides a powerful illustration of the representational dynamics described here. Discussions of *She*'s engagement with the "Woman Question" have not explicitly considered the workings of age—a surprising oversight given Ayesha's apparent immortality and the proximity of anxieties concerning women's age to their changing political and cultural status.[14] Noting that Haggard's novel was published the same year as Queen Victoria's Golden Jubilee, Adrienne Munich writes that *She* "could fittingly be considered an ominous literary monument to Victoria after fifty years of her reign" (198), a claim that, in the wake of Karen Chase's recent work, now asks readers to consider how Victoria's older age might further inflect such representations. Like Godwin's St. Leon, Ayesha is an "odd blend" of human temporal states as well, a reconstitution of the counterfeit youth that serves as the *fin de siècle*'s stamp of cultural decline in realist and gothic registers alike.

Like Vivie, Ayesha removes herself from the circuit of reproductivity. At first, Ayesha's immunity from time's arrow prevents her from consummating her sexual relationship with the mortal Leo/Kallikrates; nevertheless, the gothic imperative of Haggard's novel lays bare the abject consequences of such subversive female subjectivity. Stepping into the Spirit of the Flame to prepare for her nuptials, *She* concludes with an astonishing revelation of Ayesha's true form: the beautiful, mobile, would-be ruler and conqueror of England is stripped down to reveal nothing but a wizened primate: "Smaller she grew, and smaller yet, till she was no larger than a monkey. Now the skin was puckered into a million wrinkles, and on the shapeless face was the stamp of unutterable age" (Haggard 261–262). As if to invoke the final sentence of Darwin's *The Descent of Man* (1871)—"Man still bears in his bodily frame the indelible *stamp* of his lowly origin" (619, emphasis added)—in Haggard's novel the shocking stamp of age is the concealed reality of the counterfeit woman. *She*'s vision of individual and cultural degeneration reanimates John Donne's smearing of such "ape-leaders" three centuries earlier: "An Ape is a ridiculous and an unprofitable Beast . . . surely nothing is more unprofitable in the Commonwealth of Nature, than they that dy old maids, because they refuse to be used to that end for which they were only made" (35). The coalescing of simian imagery around the *fin de siècle* woman is strongly indicative of a new twist on an old theme:

the perilous single woman, a species new but always aping, always already apparently old, dead-set on leading others to the same sterile fate.

These examples illustrate how literary modes ranging from parody, to realism, to naturalism, and the gothic are meaningfully engaged with an unmistakable constellation of signs pertaining to gender and aging. Counterfeit youth and the senile culture it signifies therefore constitutes an important and underexplored trope in a range of disciplinary discourses concerning aging at the end of the nineteenth century. I should, however, distinguish between the notion of the counterfeit I am employing here and that of *masquerade*, an apparently analogous term that has been employed in critical discussions of age and aging. In her influential essay "Youth as Masquerade," age theorist and literary critic Kathleen Woodward traces the ways in which masquerade operates as a code of behavior that signals the primacy of youth, most obviously through the use of cosmetics, hair dye and cosmetic surgery. Woodward convincingly argues that youthfulness as masquerade, the "ideal of games and masks" first theorized in the context of feminism by Joan Riviere, "conceals and reveals and tells a certain truth of its own. Thus unconscious desire, which is mixed with castration anxiety, speaks through masquerade as symptom" (Woodward, *Discontents* 154). Woodward argues that this phenomenon underpins Aschenbach's "aging body-in-masquerade" portrayed in Mann's *Death in Venice* (1912), where "[t]he aging body is to be literally effaced—at least on the surface" (163). In the context of nineteenth-century literature, there is a long list of aging men and women alike who effect masquerade in this way: consider the beribboned Mrs. Vincy in *Middlemarch*, or Sir Walter Elliot's extreme youth-consciousness in Austen's *Persuasion*.[15]

So it is important to differentiate between the dynamics of youthful masquerade and the complex interplay between youth and the imposition of an aged, "oldening," and (in its extreme) senilized identity that is at stake in my discussion here. Youth as masquerade is inextricably implicated in the subject's desire to participate in patriarchal strictures of youthful beauty; what this chapter investigates, by contrast, is a class of *fin de siècle* subjects that are understood to somehow embody, or resemble, a clear kind of non-youth or oldened state. While related to youth as masquerade in that it too is convolved with matters of authenticity, the counterfeit youth that structures the *fin de siècle* aesthetics of senility nevertheless operates according a very different set of signals, involves a dissimilar subject and spectator, and, most essentially, entails greater repercussions that speak to the fate of species.[16] Counterfeit youth, as we have seen, is hatched within femininized subjectivities suspicious of, or even hostile to, the patriarchal foundations of women's time; the senilized subject it gives rise to embodies the possibility of a life-course narrative that rejects the fastening of life-time to the heteronormative chronology of matrimony and childbearing.

As Jack Halberstam has argued, "Queer subcultures produce alternative temporalities by allowing their participants to believe that their futures can be imagined according to logics that lie outside of the conventional forward-moving narratives of birth, marriage, reproduction, and death" ("Temporalities," n.p.). *Fin de siècle* engagements with the counterfeit subject of senility indicate an intriguing interface with queer theory around these points. Like the ideologically ambiguous motif of alchemy discussed in chapter 1, the counterfeit is necessarily a paradoxical sign of the refusal of futurity. Whether such refusal is deemed necessary or pathological—that is, whether it promises "success" of either the ideological or biological sort—is not unambiguously represented. Whether or not the counterfeit woman is capable of actualizing an effectively subversive identity on her own terms, or whether she remains a screen for the projected fears of compromised futurity, is similarly equivocal. Counterfeit subjects—queer and queering as they are—are ideally deployed in the critique of progress and its constellation of principles. The literary imagination therefore presents ideal testing ground for the polysemous ironies of progress characterized by senile subjects at the *fin de siècle*.

In an especially bombastic outburst, the opening lines of Nordau's *Degeneration* (1895) ridicule the tendency to project an overtly human narrative of aging onto the temporal entity known as the nineteenth century:

> Only the brain of a child or of a savage could form the clumsy idea that the century is a kind of living being, born like a beast or a man, passing through all the stages of existence, gradually ageing and declining after blooming childhood, joyous youth, and vigorous maturity, to die with the expiration of the hundredth year, after being afflicted in its last decade with all the infirmities of mournful senility. (1)

If readers can look beyond Nordau's turgid rhetoric, however, it is difficult to dismiss the reality of the impulse he describes. As I have argued throughout this book, British nineteenth-century literature seems indelibly (if somewhat unconsciously) structured by frameworks of inheritance, maturation, and aging more generally. Changing ideas about aging and late life themselves accrued a conceptual topography whose mid-century intensification was countered by the discernible degradations of its final decade. Clumsy as it may have seemed to some, the nineteenth century's own age stamp was supremely legible to a range of British writers at this time. Thomas Hardy's "The Darkling Thrush" (originally titled "By the Century's Deathbed, 1900"), published in his second collection, *Poems of the Past and the Present* (1901), is perhaps the most succinct instantiation of senile topography in the British writing of this period. Incorporating a suite of literal and figurative icons of aging into a bleak new-year's scene ("The ancient pulse of germ and birth / Was shrunken hard and dry," lines 13–14), Hardy's speaker reads in "The land's sharp features . . . / The Century's corpse outleant" (9–10). The poem's only vital sign is both a reflection and a refraction of the exhausted century's terrestrial state: "An aged thrush, frail, gaunt, and small, / In blast-beruffled plume, / Had chosen thus to fling his soul / Upon the growing gloom" (21–24). Charles E. May has read this poem as a rejoinder to Keats's vernal Nightingale, concluding that Hardy inverts Keats's Romantic view of Nature to render it "absurd" (65). Perhaps, but: in light of what I have described as the fin-de-siècle's senile topography, different emphases materialize. Like Rhoda's "inscrutable" interaction with Monica's infant child (Gissing 332), Hardy's senescent figure of the new year is the "caroling" [sic] embodiment of prolonged degradation (25). The apparent paradox becomes less contradictory by reading such figures through the *fin de siècle*'s aesthetics of senility: as beings new but old, as signals of a speculative, inscrutable progress whose issue—hopeful or otherwise—is the germ of an unreadable epoch to come.

This chapter has described how certain *fin de siècle* subjects were conceived via temporal narratives inconsistent with the traditional circumscriptions of conventional (often heteronormative) narratives of life-course. Such new and destabilizing subjects—especially emergent classes of non-reproductive women—were regularly identified by means of hermeneutical tactics no longer able to tie women's life-course to traditional categories of wife and mother. Just as the faltering institution of marriage and the eroding claims of imperial progress seemed to give birth to beings likewise in their dotage, *fin de siècle* writing regularly employed pathologically oldened subjects (odd women, the aged child or *puer senex*, and so on) as vehicles for exploring innovative fears of the new. Consistent with what I have called the longevity narrative, counterfeit youth and the pathologized, ironic progress of species it implies makes legible a broader cultural concern with senility at the *fin de siècle:* namely, that it signifies both an individualized type of degeneration and population-based corruption of the forward-looking narrative of Britain's future. By taking this position, I contend that "senility"—today as medically obsolete a term as its contemporary condition "hysteria" and exclusively a stigmatizing slur—can nevertheless be deployed as an aesthetically productive concept within the context of literary Age Studies: as an amalgam of youth and older age distinct from the "masquerade" that critics have invoked in discussions of literary representations of age and aging. One salient moment in medical history encapsulates this last facet of the aesthetics of senescence I have been describing. In 1901, hundreds of miles away, a hitherto undistinguished German doctor would encounter a fifty-one-year-old woman with an anomalous set of symptoms: acute memory loss, disorientation, hallucinations, and pronounced psychosocial incompetence. Louis Alzheimer's first recorded case marks a provocative convergence of literary and medicalized re-presentations of aging: the patient, Auguste D, the first of an incipient population that would come to signify a new and distinctly pathologized embodiment of older age. By the end of the nineteenth century, there could be no question that senescence was not only an ideologically fraught state of being, but an aesthetically prolific marker as well—one that marked the end of an epoch, a new figure of oblivion, a future for subject and species that promised anew the old words: *sans everything.*

Chapter 5

Writing Twenty-First-Century Aging Populations

Looking back over the five preceding chapters, clearly *what it is to grow old*—to borrow Matthew Arnold's phrasing—was a pressing question for nineteenth-century British literature, philosophy, economics, science, and medicine alike. Without denying that life's greener days, rituals, and narratives still occupied a significant share of the literary imagination, I have argued that the tendency to perceive aging as a collective, social issue over the course of the long nineteenth century added a decidedly new dimension to the moral and theological lineaments that had governed ideations of later life since at least the early modern period. Contrast, for example, the optimistic accumulations of Robert Browning's often-cited "Rabbi Ben Ezra" (1864)—"Grow old along with me! / The best is yet to be" (1–2)—and that of Alfred Tennyson's perpetually aging Tithonus (1833, revised 1859), whose immortality does not spare him the debilities of the fourth age. Or indeed, Arnold's forceful conclusion to "Growing Old," published when he was in his mid-forties:

> It is—last stage of all—
> When we are frozen up within, and quite
> The phantom of ourselves,
> To hear the world applaud the hollow ghost
> Which blamed the living man. (35–40)

Browning's untroubled because recuperative ideal of aging—where the real or perceived losses of older age are compensated for by gains in other quarters such as wealth, wisdom, and experience—is contradicted by Arnold's tragic sketch of the evacuation of selfhood in late life. Gesturing toward the Aristotelian association of old age, cold, and lethargy, Arnold's senescent "phantom" is "frozen up within": a vacant mass of dense, emotional frigidity, far removed from the ardently animating passions of youth. In its strange double vision of emptiness and surfeit, Arnold's "hollow ghost" transforms the individual catastrophe of old age into a social spectacle. (Such bleak descriptors continue to echo in present-day imagery of older persons, particularly those with dementia, who may be viewed—often by their loved ones—as empty shells of their former selves.) To grow old is no longer to occupy the crowning stage of life's journey, as it did for Browning's Rabbi. Instead, the horrors of the fourth age implicate the destiny of a population (the anonymous beholding "world") beyond the individual sufferer ("the living man").

As we have seen, what constituted "oldness" over the course of the nineteenth century ranged from externally perceptible bodily features and behaviors to far more nuanced phenomena, resonances, and subterranean associations. Alongside the confining structure of the "stages" model, which architected individual life as a series of successive age roles and phases, there emerged a discernible sense of age as a conditional state: one far more reflective of affective and conditional (often social) relationships that were themselves subject to change and alteration—one might say, to aging. What I have called the longevity narrative reflects this shifting emplotment of life-course by conceptualizing age, aging, and lifespan in relationship to the massified context of population. Importantly, the emergence of the longevity narrative is not necessarily tied to a celebratory or emancipatory view of life-course. To recast old age as a state is to recognize that nineteenth-century British representations of senescence were more likely than their predecessors to regard age and aging as a comparably open, even nomadic condition of being: one thoroughly entangled with newly age-oriented interests of extra-literary disciplines like medicine, philosophy, and economics.

This new materialization of senescence affects how we read old age and aging in the nineteenth-century British novel. If life-course is conceptualized simply as a succession of inverted stages (as it traditionally has been, from the *Bildungs*-ascent of youth to the analogous decline of later life), then we are left without the means to critically interpret phenomena—real or imagined, "lived," speculative, or fictional—that confound notions of chronological progression: rejuvenation, not looking or feeling one's age, generational discontinuity, the *puer senex* or aged child, to name just a few. The readings I offer in this book locate aging and later life within a constellation of emergent concepts—including ephebiphobia, frail Romanticism, waste and repair, senile topographies, capacity, and containment—that were more or less consciously deployed to make new sense of human aging throughout this period. In her essay "The Problem of Theory" (1999), Elizabeth Grosz writes that concepts are "always and only occasioned by problems," and function as "temporary contraptions" that provoke "multiple responses, conceptual, perceptual, and affective." The entanglement of aging with paradox and paradoxical thinking throughout this book is an index of this very multiplicity. In "Growing Old," Arnold's disruptive syntax—"Yes, this, and more; but not / Ah, 'tis not what in youth we dreamed [age] 'twould be!" (11–12)—fittingly distills this truth to its textual essence. Aging is never this or that alone, as Arnold knew. Recognizing the essentially paradoxical nature of aging helps clarify why its intellectual examination in the past, and the present, so often involves accommodating potentially contradictory arguments and conceptualizations. For even though our oldening is shared, universal, we nevertheless endure in our aging alone, solitary phantoms.

The stakes of this new, double-stranded vision of life are particularly suited for exploration by the literary imagination. The texts I have considered in this book demonstrate how the tenses and heteroglossia of fiction help mediate very real, embodied states of age and their representation within the complex, textualized temporalities of the novel. As a final case study, I briefly turn to Anthony Trollope's notorious dystopian novel, *The Fixed Period* (1881–2), the last published during his lifetime, and the convergence of key concerns regarding aging with his *Autobiography* (published posthumously in 1883). On the one hand, *The Fixed Period* dramatizes the demographic construction of older age as a catastrophic force; set in 1980, it imagines a fictional British colony, Britannula, where euthanasia is made compulsory at the age of 67-and-one-half. Not unlike William Godwin's negotiation of philosophical and literary portraits of immortality, almost a century later Trollope's overtly fictional exploration of aging presents a multi-genre exposition of the author's aging body as it is rendered in a decidedly less speculative text. Intriguingly, Trollope wrote this novel in bad health in the year before his death—at the age of sixty-seven and eight months, no less. It is perpetually unclear whether Trollope intended his work as make-believe; his letters written at this time betray acute irritation with his own failing health, and of his novel he allegedly claimed, "It's all true—I mean every word of it."[1] As I have argued in detail elsewhere (2012), in its obsessive attention to numbers and statistics *The Fixed Period* registers accelerating anxieties about an aging population. Read alongside Trollope's *Autobiography*, it sketches a direct line of association between the perceived problems of an aging population and that of the aging writer.

The Fixed Period overtly depicts aging as a critical issue of demographic containment and, more specifically, in the terms of what scholars have recently called "apocalyptic demography" (Cruikshank 27). As the reformist President John Neverbend explains, "Statistics have told us that the sufficient sustenance of an old man is more costly than the feeding of a young one. . . . Statistics also have told us that the unprofitable young and the no less unprofitable old form a third of the population" (11). To contain the ballooning cost and numbers associated with the aged, Neverbend passes a popular law concerning "the prearranged ceasing to live of those who would otherwise become old" (10). Behind this euphemistic veil, the Fixed Period law is specifically one of containment: temporally, in its limitation of life to 67.5 years, but also spatially, for the law demands that the elderly spend their last year in Necropolis, a seraphic college spatially zoned off from the rest of society so as to enhance the palatability of "depositing" the aged. Such containment is necessary, Neverbend confides, because of "an ill-judged and a thoughtless tenderness" that has forced the aged "to live a useless and painful life" (11). He addresses the reader directly: "Look round on the men whom you can remember, and tell me, on how many of them life has not sat as a burden at seventy years of age?" (36–37). Neverbend's sympathy for the individual bearer of years quickly slides toward anxieties for the wellbeing of the non-old. He personifies the nation by conceiving it as a noble beast staggering under the weight of so many years, so many old people: "How are a people to thrive when so weighted?" (11). Under the Fixed Period system, the elderly "would depart with the full respect of all their fellow-citizens. To how many does that lot now fall?" (12). Yet ensuring the dignified departure of the elderly would have further civic benefits. Overwhelmed by "the idleness of years that are useless," Neverbend complains that "our bridges, our railways, our Government are not provided for. Our young men are again becoming torpid beneath the weight imposed upon them" (14). Neverbend makes a express appeal to those reading his memoir: "Let the reader think of the burden"—the twin burden suffered, but also exerted, by the weight of age and an elderly population (11).

The aged body—in both its individual and its demographically conceived senses—becomes for Neverbend a cipher of cost. As the frank Mrs. Neverbend steadily insists, however, the capitalist aims behind the Fixed Period are indistinguishable from its humanitarian artifice: a tastefully ornamented college will only ensure that "all the old men and women may be killed artistically" (94). Mrs. Neverbend's gesture toward aesthetics is not frivolous. For as much as John Neverbend is the statistically minded author of the Fixed Period policy, he is also the writer of this fictional memoir. The reader first encounters Neverbend aboard the John Bright, having been politely removed from Britannula by Captain Battleax and deported to England. Now sixty years old, Neverbend is struck with a desire to "publish . . . a book in which I should declare my theory—this very book which I have so nearly brought to a close" (175). It is significant that Neverbend is able to so fluidly transition between demographic and writerly presentations of his Fixed Period cause; indeed, following his current publication, Neverbend determines to write yet another volume as "argumentative and statistical, as I have here been fanciful, though true to details" (195).

Were Neverbend merely a satirical exercise, it is unlikely his laments would overlap so conspicuously with Trollope's anxiously quantified reporting of his lifelong productivity. Without wholly espousing the principles presented in his dystopian fiction experiment, Trollope's *Autobiography* confides nevertheless, "I have prided myself especially in completing [my work] within the proposed time,—and I have always done so. There has ever been the record before me, and a week passed with an insufficient number of pages has been a blister to my eye, and a month so disgraced would have been a sorrow to my heart" (chapter 7). Read alongside his strange fictional meditation on the enforced containment of lifespan, the *Autobiography* highlights a private struggle between writing too little and too much. "[I have] never put a book out of hand short of the number by a single word," writes Trollope, "I may also say that the excess has been very small. I have prided myself on completing my work exactly within the proposed dimensions" (chapter 7). The speculative exercise of imagining aging is, in Trollope's case, intimately related to his materially embodied identity as a novelist, further entangling *The Fixed Period*'s speculative politics with the life of the aging author. In keeping with the paradoxical thinking that so often characterizes nineteenth-century portraits of aging, in Trollope's case it is difficult to assess where the fearsome account of population aging is distinct from similarly grave assessments of chronological agedness. Like Gissing's *The Odd Women* and the social crises its demographically defined characters pointed to, both Trollope's *The Fixed Period* and *Autobiography* present aging into later life as a matter of social containment constantly threatened by catastrophe. Be it chronological agedness or, as we saw in chapter 4, the senile symbolics of human excess, by the late nineteenth century it was possible to imagine society's collapse under the strain of too many years, too many people.

The Fixed Period is one of several late-nineteenth-century British novels that imagine a socially disruptive aging population. The shared thematics of Samuel Butler's *Erewhon; Or, Over the Range* (1872), Walter Besant's *The Inner House* (1888), and Lillian Frances Mentor's *The Day of Resis* (1897) presage the ways the nascent reality of population aging disturbed the narrative unity of an individual life where old age might have once constituted a quiescent dénouement. This new temporal disjointedness—realized in its extreme form by the *fin de siècle* nightmare of counterfeit youth and the senile subject—provided the conceptual and aesthetic conditions of possibility for later literary experimentations with non-processional nature of human aging. F. Scott Fitzgerald's *The Curious Case of Benjamin Button* (1922), Gertrude Atherton's *Black Oxen* (1923), C.P. Snow's *New Lives for Old* (1932), and Aldous Huxley's *After Many a Summer* (1939) were just a few examples of Anglophone modernism that experimented textually with the temporal and narrative tethers of older age. More recently, Chris Buckley's *Boomsday* (2007) provides an up-to-the-minute rehash of *The Fixed Period*'s plot (Trollope's novel is itself an update of Middleton's early-seventeenth-century play *The Old Law*), wherein "voluntary transitioning"—a Neverbendian euphemism for elder suicide—is proposed as a means of solving American Social Security insolvency. Kazuo Ishiguro's *Never Let Me Go* (2005) and Gary Shteyngart's *Super Sad True Love Story* (2010) likewise locate their textual experiments in the proximal future as a method of working through their respective engagements with "demographic demagoguery" (to use Margaret Cruikshank's term, 27). With its Flaubertian intertextual scaffolding, Minae Mizumura's decidedly more realist *Inheritance From Mother* (2012; translated from Japanese in 2017) further suggests the insinuation of a globally recognizable thematics of aging and ageism, perhaps even the emergence of a transnational canon of aging pop(ulation) literature.

Brief excursions into the present aside, *The Aesthetics of Senescence* is temporally bounded by war: beginning, more or less, with the French Revolution's backlash against the *ancien régime*, and concluding shortly before what Wilfred Owen would describe as the "shrill, demented choirs of wailing shells" that began falling in 1914. Of course, diverse forms of extreme imperial violence enabled the very existence of British Empire over the course of the nineteenth century. One of the obvious limitations of this book is its focus on the geographical limits of Great Britain and, more specifically still, England, as opposed to the various iterations of aging that undoubtedly shaped a national literary tradition steeped in colonial networks of appropriation and dispossession. Nevertheless, in writing this study of the relatively recent past, an Age Studies approach has taught me to attend closely to the apparent incompatibility of age cohorts as a kind of quiet bellwether. In the searching query that opens "Anthem for Doomed Youth" (1917)—"What passing-bells for these who die as cattle?"—Owen's age-configured representation of the First World War is a fitting peal for this population unknowingly born predestined for an early and ignoble encounter with a traumatically massified expression of senescence (line 7). When it surfaces as a theme, content, and aspect of literary form, age becomes a tactic for sensing emergent crises of sociality. The speculative potential of fiction and literature more broadly creates the space needed to examine the appearance of aging as a cipher of risk, crisis, and impending social calamity. Whether such crises are real or perceived is in many ways beside the point.

The temporal and geographical specificities of this book bear a certain semblance to our own time. As Anna Kornbluh and Benjamin Morgan astutely observe, "ours is also a gilded age of income inequality, of financial speculation, of de facto debtor's prisons, of capitalist exploitation, of global inequity, of misplaced faith in evolutionary psychology, of widespread reliance on coal-based energy" (n.p.). To this list I would add the renewed statistical panic of surplus populations, aging ones particularly. Contemporary media, medicine, and economics regularly frame aging as nothing less than an imminent social catastrophe, while other conclusions (like taking population aging as a public health success or the outcome of improved medical care) have been overwhelmed entirely. As we collectively age into the late days of the anthropocene—itself a nineteenth-century British innovation—crises of resource sharing and culpability for their mismanagement have been thoroughly scaffolded by "adversarial ageism" (Harvie 2018) and cohort-conscious narratives of intergenerational catastrophe. Importantly, it is not just the material reality of an increased proportion of older persons in society that has returned (or indeed, never really gone away); it is the way that demography has catalyzed increasingly dire pronouncements about the endgame of Western society itself. Whether there exists the possibility of some sort of *rapprochement*, as Mary Shelley so tenuously imagined in *The Last Man* (1826), will be evident soon enough.

From the vantage point of a twenty-first-century reader, *The Aesthetics of Senescence* offers a new perspective on the social figuration of age and aging in Romantic and Victorian literature. The long life of the Godwin-Malthus debate affirms that nineteenth-century culture found itself increasingly in conflict over matters of age. If we consider the lasting imprint of Malthus's *Essay* upon the Victorian period—its influence upon the 1832 Poor Laws, or its well-documented prompting of Alfred Wallace's and Charles Darwin's theorization of natural selection—then surely it is remarkable that the matters of age and aging are not more prevalent in critical assessments of this period. Just as the *Essay*'s future-oriented logic of population looks askance at youth's sanguinity, so does the Romantic youth model regard the stagnant past. This apparent impasse allows us to glimpse an important generalization concerning the biopolitics of aging as well. The preservation of the past—be it as a more or less Burkean or gerontocratic ideal, or in the bodily state of youth itself—fruitlessly wishes to retain in perpetuity that which is destined to change. Given the anti-aging paradigm of our own day, contemporary readers might already sense that so long as any age-identified cohort carries ideopathological connotations or is maligned as some sort of social ill, the biopolitics of aging are always conservative.

In writing this book, my goal has been to acknowledge, if only partially investigate, the multiplicity of relations that make "age" a meaningful analytical category, for singular and plural subjects alike. No longer can we entertain fictions of the singular human life extracted from a larger networked assemblage of relations, be they human, historical, or the infinite otherwise. As outlined in my introduction, this book has demonstrated the ways that more diverse models of age, aging, and later life were in circulation throughout the nineteenth century; I have no doubt that there are more, and more still to come as the limits of human lifespan continue to entrance the labors of science, medicine, and literature alike.

As I was writing this conclusion, I happened upon a fragment of a poem that I had never read before:

> Obsessed, bewildered
>
> By the shipwreck
> Of the singular
>
> We have chosen the meaning
> Of being numerous.

"Of Being Numerous," the forty-part title poem of George Oppen's 1968 eponymous collection, describes a series of apparently mundane civic scenes in New York City. A powerful meditation on the necessity of intersubjective being, crystallized in the seventh stanza I cite above, it also weaves into its catalogue a partisan intergenerational gambit: "For the people of that flow / Are new, the old / New to age as the young / To youth" (stanza 4). Oppen's poem speaks to me for the way it captures the essential conflict between individual and collective identities at the heart of my study, and for its provocative renewal of why we might—must, even—choose to age with, rather than against, our numerousness. At this point it seems fair to conclude that we have never been intergenerational: the "shipwreck / of the singular" is not merely the awful endgame of Western individualism. It also names a chronic, ongoing, perhaps incurable insufficiency to imagine the plural subjectivies—reduced by Arnold to "hollow ghosts"—that exist outside our own cohort identity.

What's left, it seems to me, is to use the productive power of paradox that sits at the core of this book as an ethic of living: to do all we can to write, work, and live in the service of the future perfect, of that which will have one day already been so. Literature's capacity to accommodate and nourish such paradoxical thinking makes it an ideal forum for testing out the complexities of aging and its representations; it is also, in contrast to the objectives of other disciplinary traditions, the very hallmark of literary ways of knowing. To amass a partisan knowledge from these literary experiments—their failures, inadequacies, lateness, and prospects for living—is to me the reason we might choose to shape a life-course by reading. As writers of the past knew very well, we can only speculate as to where aging takes us from here. Written in 1816, Percy Bysshe Shelley's "Alastor; or, The Spirit of Solitude" concludes with the knowledge that "Nature's vast frame, the web of human things, / Birth and the grave . . . are not as they were." Two centuries later, the precarious reality of markedly longer human lifespans means that what we suppose to be the human condition requires similar recalibration. For lives numerous and singular alike, the futures of aging are as clear as the night sky. We will never again be as we once were.

Notes

Introduction

1. Thomas Robert Malthus, *An Essay on the Principle of Population and A Summary View of the Principle of Population*, edited by Philip Appleman, Norton, 1976. Unless otherwise noted, all references to the *Essay* are to this reprint of the original 1798 edition—since Malthus makes important revisions to the *Essay*'s argument, structure, and forms of evidence in his later editions (in 1803, 1806, 1807, 1817, and 1826). In the Appendix to the 1806 edition, for instance, he attempts to clarify his position by claiming, "I am not an enemy to population; I am an enemy to vice and misery" (see "Appendix, 1806" in *An Essay on the Principle of Population*, edited by Donald Winch). This might modulate the mistaken view of Malthus as a callous apologist for the wretched state of the poor; but in later editions, it is difficult to argue against the author as an enemy of youth, as well as of vice and misery. In later years, Malthus still cleaves to his original ideological nexus of vice, misery, and the reproductive capacity of youth first articulated in 1798.

2. References to "massification" invoke George Lukács's Hegelian-Marxist account of population as one of the defining experiences of nineteenth-century life. See McLane; Steinlight; James Chandler (42); and Lukács, *The Historical Novel* (24).

3. In a chapter of his *Archaeologies* titled "Longevity as Class Struggle," Fredric Jameson describes George Bernard Shaw's 1918–1920 play *Back to Methuselah* as an "immortality or longevity drama" (331). The distinction between Jameson's appellation and mine is obvious: my goal is to map how developments in the nineteenth-century novel match the changing concepts of senescence and life-course. More specifically, I examine how the novel challenges the longstanding metaphor of age as a stage. (I also view Jameson's version of "longevity" as closer to Gruman's idea of prolongevity—"the significant extension of life by human action" [3]—rather than as a reconceptualization of senescence itself.) Speaking of *Back to Methuselah*, Jameson concludes that "the longevity drama is not 'really' about longevity at all, but rather about something else, which can a little more rapidly be identified as

History" (335). My own definition of the longevity narrative—while it inevitably includes broader concerns such as temporality—is very much about refiguring old age within a model of life that encompasses not just individuals, but populations.

4. Data regarding population growth are drawn from multiple authoritative sources, including Wrigley and Schofield, Thane's "Social Histories of Old Age and Ageing," and "Historical Statistics on Population for the Country" (*A Vision of Britain through Time* initiative), which draws its statistical tables from British Census data beginning in 1801.

5. This range reflects slight variations reflected in British Census data entries (see "Historical Statistics" [Rate: Percentage Aged over 65], Wrigley and Schofield [217], and Ottaway [22]). Wrigley and Schofield also note, and correct for, a widely acknowledged tendency of elderly to exaggerate age in early-nineteenth-century census data (see 109–111).

6. This classed difference in life expectancy persisted throughout the century, as Antonovsky describes. "Vital Statistics of Families in the Upper and Professional Classes," published in *the Journal of the Royal Statistical Society* (1874), states that for the current year, "the expectation of life at birth in the upper and professional classes was 53 years indicating an advantage of about 10 years over the expectation for the general population" (C. Ansell, in Antonovsky 35).

7. As reported by Statistics Canada (2016); United States data from Census Bureau "Age & Sex Tables" (2016); and United Kingdom data from Office for National Statistics (2011).

8. For more on the realities of poverty, old age, and gender in nineteenth-century England, see Goose.

9. In full: *The General History of China Containing a Geographical, Historical, Chronological, Political and Physical Description of the Empire of China, Chinese-Tartary, Corea, and Thibet; Including an Exact and Particular Account of Their Customs, Manners, Ceremonies, Religion, Arts, and Sciences: The Whole Adorn'd with Curious Maps, and Variety of Copper-Plates*. The book had a significant impact on European society, and was quickly translated into most European languages and added to academic libraries.

10. During the American Revolution, scholars used such generational tropes to grapple with the implications of a conflict that was at once civil and imperial (see Fliegelman). Similar anxieties have been repeated throughout history ever since. In 1920s France and Britain, Pat Thane writes, "The combination of rapidly falling birth-rates and lengthening life-expectancy in a period when there was a perceived military threat from apparently 'younger' countries, in particular Germany, and a perceived cultural threat from the growth of non-white populations in other continents, produced in France and Britain doom-laden predictions from demographers and social scientists about the social conservatism and economic, imperial and military decline which was anticipated, as these nations lost their youthful vitality" ("Social Histories," 96).

11. For a discussion of these comments see Patricia James, especially 100–101.

12. See McDonagh, "Infanticidal Mothers and Dead Babies" 11–20. For an analysis of Malthusian themes in Gaskell's novel *Cranford*, see Niles.

13. "Ancient" is a word and concept that Burke was very fond of. Paley calls the term a "key word" throughout *Reflections* (see *Apocalypse and Millennium in English Romantic Poetry* 49).

14. See Steven Blakemore's "Burke and the Fall of Language." Blakemore argues that Burke consciously appropriates and adapts Cicero's text to position himself as the "Cato of England" (51).

15. See entries for United Nations (2017), World Health Organization (2018), National Institutes of Health (2016), and World Bank (2017).

16. For an overview of recent calls for "strategic presentism," see "Manifesto of the V21 Collective: Ten Theses" and the "V21 Forum on Strategic Presentism."

Chapter 1

1. Hereafter referred to as *Political Justice* (*PJ*), and cited parenthetically throughout by volume and page number of the 1798 edition. Critics have consistently linked Godwin's fiction to his philosophical writings, although their assessments of its fidelity to the tenets of *Political Justice* are somewhat inconsistent. See Rounce, Kelly, Handwerk for more on Godwin's own responses to *Political Justice* in his later career.

2. Hereafter abbreviated as "Of Health." On the first page of *Godwin's Political Justice*, Mark Philp acknowledges the difficulties voiced by Godwin's critics concerning the question of prolonged life and immortality. Although Philp goes on to situate Godwin's philosophical project within the particular British intellectual context of 1790s Dissent, "Of Health, and the Prolongation of Human Life" is not discussed. Literary analyses of *St. Leon* and Godwin's work more generally (including those by Clemit, Chandler, Von Schlun, and Collings) make little to no reference to "Of Health."

3. Although Ni Chonaill makes no mention of *St. Leon*, she does argue that "rather than reading Godwin's conjectures on earthly immortality as a rational idea, they are more accurately understood as an ideological climax to his perfectibilist philosophy. In this way, they emerge more clearly as one aspect of the secular ambitions of human progress which, as a philosophy, intended to transfer utopian concepts of paradise and immortality from the realm of religion to the earthly domain" (39).

4. See Mark Philp's *Godwin's Political Justice* and Priestley's variorum edition of Godwin's *Enquiry Concerning Political Justice* (vol. 3).

5. Godwin's idea that it might eventually be possible to eliminate the need for sleep is consistent with his speculations about prolonged life. His initial statements from the 1793 version may be condensed into this: "Before death can be banished, we must banish sleep, death's image" (see volume three of Priestley's

edition of Godwin's text for his critical introduction and notes, which provide a full delineation of variant readings across all three of Godwin's versions). These comments were removed for the 1796 and 1798 versions. In the final edition, the only statement about sleep reads: "When reason resigns the helm, and our ideas fluctuate without order or direction, we sleep" (*PJ* 2:522).

6. In *The English Jacobin Novel, 1780–1805*, Kelly identifies Godwin's psychological realism as the feature that distinguishes him from other Jacobin writers associated with eighteenth-century philosophical discourses of human psychology—notably Jacobin novelist Robert Bage. "It is this difference which places Bage at the end of the eighteenth century and Godwin at the beginning of the nineteenth, Bage as a product of the Enlightenment and Godwin as a forerunner of Romanticism" (17).

7. Godwin's Humean turn has been noted by a number of scholars. For a representative example, see James Chandler's *England in 1819*, 522 n. 28. Mark Philp makes note of Godwin's "resist[ance]" to "Humean conclusions" on p. 146 of *Godwin's Political Justice* but concedes Godwin's "move towards the ethical theories of Hume, Smith and Butler" (147) on the pages that follow.

8. Referring to Godwin, and briefly to other writers about prolonged life such as Hufeland, Cabanis, and Condorcet, Marie Mulvey-Roberts writes that after "the Scientific Revolution, the Enlightenment had redrawn the boundaries of knowledge and redefined the material and moral universe. The pursuit of immortality formed part of this revised epistemology, making thinkers now more inclined to question the limits of mortality" (*Gothic* 30).

9. In his encomium to Godwin in *Spirit of the Age: Or, Contemporary Portraits* (1824), William Hazlitt writes "No work in our time gave such a blow to the philosophical mind of the country as the celebrated *Enquiry Concerning Political Justice*. Tom Paine was considered for the time as a Tom Fool to him; Paley an old woman; Edmund Burke a flashy sophist. Truth, moral truth, it was supposed, had here taken up its abode; and these were the oracles of thought. 'Throw aside your books of chemistry,' said Wordsworth to a young man, a student in the Temple, 'and read Godwin on Necessity.'" James Chandler also includes this anecdote in his *England in 1819* (508).

10. In *The Coming of Age*, Simone de Beauvoir writes, "All men are mortal. . . . A great many of them become old: almost none ever foresees this state before it is upon him" (4). My argument proposes that the medicalized and politicized connotations of age in Godwin's work indicate the emergence of a newly conditional figuration of the "state"—one very different from the metaphor of a dramatized stage of life, filled with inevitable roles.

11. In his essay "Erasmus Darwin and the Fungus School" (2002), Alan Richardson notes that members of the Johnson circle like William Godwin and Mary Wollstonecraft "are generally seen as espousing an associationist, social constructivist view of mind" against which they defined the dangerously reductive arguments of

physiological and scientific "materialists." However, Richardson suggests that Godwin's quiet materialism—that is, his alignment with Erasmus Darwin's views on reproduction and the advancement of species—emerges in his reversal in *St. Leon* of the individualism he espouses in *Political Justice*.

12. See Thomas R. Cole's essential *The Journey of Life: A Cultural History of Aging in America*.

13. Historians of Age Studies have provided admirable surveys of the medical and philosophical texts on aging available since the classical period. A selective list might include Cole, Gerald J. Gruman's *A History of Ideas about the Prolongation of Life*, and Helen Small's *The Long Life*. For a more specialized historical study focused on Britain, see Susannah Ottaway's *The Decline of Life: Old Age in Eighteenth-Century England*. Steven Marx's *Youth Against Age: Generational Strife in Renaissance Poetry* provides a very useful historical-literary account of prevalent topoi and motifs associated with aging in the early modern period.

14. I thank Christine Lehleiter at the University of Toronto for this reference and translation.

15. Hufeland's *The Art of Prolonging Life* was translated and published in 1797 by John Bell of London (the word *Makrobiotic*, then a newcomer to the language, was added to the title for the third edition of 1805). Hufeland is most commonly credited with popularizing Jenner's smallpox vaccination in his homeland (see Aschoff). The most detailed description of Hufeland's work on aging is Gerald J. Gruman's *A History of Ideas about the Prolongation of Life*. Hufeland is also briefly mentioned in several books, including de Beauvoir's *The Coming of Age*, Cole's *The Journey of Life: A Cultural History of Aging in America*, Ottaway's *The Decline of Life: Old Age in Eighteenth-Century England*, Corkhill's "Charlatanism in Goethe's *Faust I* and Tieck's *William Lovell*," and Katz's *Disciplining Old Age: The Formation of Gerontological Knowledge* (1996). English literary studies have not yet awoken to the intriguing critical opportunities offered by Hufeland's work: he is mostly unknown, with the exception of a few brief notes on John Keats's medical context in Hermione De Almeida's *Romantic Medicine and John Keats* and his influence on Samuel Taylor Coleridge (see Vickers's *Coleridge and the Doctors 1795–1806* and Levere's *Poetry Realized in Nature: Samuel Taylor Coleridge and Early Nineteenth-Century Science*).

16. A 1798 review in *Monthly Visitor and Pocket Companion* claims, "if it were a native production, might be suspected to lead chiefly to the recommendation of some quack medicine. It is however of a very different kind, and contains a philosophical illustration of that very interesting subject"—that is, long life ("Long Life," 250). Writing in 1830, Coleridge eagerly asserted Hufeland's position among the great figures of contemporary medicine. In 1867, a second English edition of *The Art of Prolonging Life* was published (ed. Erasmus Wilson), and glowing reviews into the early years of the twentieth century included ""Hufeland's Art of Prolonging Life," *London Quarterly Review*, 2:3 (Mar. 1854), p. 293; The Art of Prolonging Life" in the *Examiner* 3573 (Jul. 1876), p. 831; J. Burney Yeo's "Long Life and How to

Attain it," *Nineteenth Century: A Monthly Review*, 23.133 (Mar. 1888), p. 370; and Jas Gault's "The Prolongation of Life," *Academy* (Jan. 1908), p. 348.

17. *The Art of Prolonging Life* was not listed among the books found in Godwin's personal library following his death in 1836 (see Godwin, *Catalogue of the curious library of that very eminent and distinguished author, William Godwin, Esq.* [etc.]). Nor does a search of Godwin's diary suggest it was among his daily readings (see *The Diary of William Godwin*). Even so, in August 1797 the physician Thomas Beddoes—like Godwin, a prominent member of Joseph Johnson's Dissenting circle—reviewed *The Art of Prolonging Life* in the *Monthly Review* 23, pp. 505–506, and his *Hygëia: or, Essays Moral and Medical On the Causes Affecting the Personal State of Our Middling and Affluent Classes* (1802) contains numerous references to Hufeland's speculations concerning extended life expectancy. Vickers concludes that Beddoes's work in pneumatic medicine in the 1790s "laid the basis for the first surgical anaesthetics in the 1840s when the anaesthetic properties of nitrous oxide were fully recognized" (see "Thomas Beddoes and the German Psychological Tradition," 319); intriguingly, Beddoes's interest in Hufeland's work also indicates his facilitating role in the increasingly medicalized understanding of old age in the early years of the nineteenth century, and suggests the proximity of such ideas to Godwin at this time.

18. In *Romantic Narrative: Shelley, Hays, Godwin, Wollstonecraft*, Tilottama Rajan identifies alchemy and gambling as "operative metaphors" (144) in Godwin's *St. Leon*, and she discusses the significance of speculation in contemporary critiques of "the mere understanding" characteristic to Common Sense philosophy (151). Despite our similar spheres of interest, Rajan takes a different approach to unpacking the function of speculation in the context of Godwin's novel, mainly by positioning speculation as the "site of a deep division between British and continental thought" (152), and then by focusing on Kant's double-edged critique of speculation as a means of grappling with his own attractions to both pure and practical reason. Where our studies overlap, however, is in a shared appreciation for the speculative foundations of the novel form itself. Readers interested in the multiple connotations of speculation during this period are encouraged to consult Rajan's *Romantic Narrative*, especially chapter 5, "Gambling, Alchemy, Speculation: Godwin's Critique of Pure Reason in *St. Leon*."

19. The full title: *Thoughts Occasioned by the Perusal of Dr. Parr's Spital Sermon, Preached at Christ Church, April 15, 1800: Being a Reply to the Attacks of Dr. Parr, Mr. Mackintosh, the Author of an Essay on Population, and Others*. Godwin's graciousness would disappear by 1820, when, in the latest edition of the *Essay*, Malthus deleted a chapter on the *Spital Sermon* to make room for a commentary on Robert Owen's *New View of Society* (Patricia James 376).

20. Despite his initial refusal, Ugolino "started groping over each; / and after they were dead, [he] called them for / two days; then fasting had more force than grief" (73–75). As punishment, Ugolino is condemned to eternally gnaw at the head of his betrayer, Ruggieri. Dante writes,

> We had already taken leave of him,
> when I saw two shades frozen in one hole,
> so that one's head served as the other's cap;
> and just as he who's hungry chews his bread,
> one sinner dug his teeth into the other
> right at the place where the brain is joined to the nape. (canto XXXII,
>   124–129)

21. Also used by Spencer and his contemporaries to refer to the ancestral matrix.

22. For example, after being wrongfully accused of attempting to seduce Charles's (aptly named) lover Pandora, St. Leon is revealed to be an alchemist and banished from his son's party. Just as he did when he was younger, Charles rejects Leon as an "execrable" (346) object and refuses to be "contaminated" (214) by his father's excessive economy of immortality: "Magic dissolves the whole principle and arrangement of human action, subverts all generous enthusiasm and dignity, and renders life itself loathsome and intolerable. Wretch that you are!" (446). Charles's speech is an infernal near-repetition of Marguerite's after she deduces that St. Leon is cheating the course of lifespan by means of the dark arts ("How unhappy the wretch, the monster rather let me say, who is without an equal" [227]). Charles scorns the "envenomed gift" (297) of eternal life—not simply because it corrupts domestic affection, but because it also scrambles biological succession.

Chapter 2

1. Other deconstructive readings have demonstrated how hegemonic binarisms, especially those linked to apparently atemporal facets of identity (male/female, occident/orient, human/animal), fail to hold under the annihilating weight of plague (see particularly Barbara Johnson or Cynthia Schoolar Williams).

2. Aristotle writes, "We must remember that an animal is by nature humid and warm, and to live is to be of such a constitution, while old age is dry and cold, and so is a corpse"; see *On Longevity and Shortness of Life*, 3. For more on "Promethean politics," see Anne Mellor's *Mary Shelley*, 70. I cite Percy Shelley's "A Defence of Poetry" in *Romantic Poetry and Prose*, 744–762.

3. Almost two decades later, Percy Bysshe Shelley would ingratiate himself with his future father-in-law by way of famously agitated dismissals of their shared nemesis—as evinced in "The Revolt of Islam" (1816) and his prefatory remarks to *Prometheus Unbound* (1820): "For my part I had rather be damned with Plato and Lord Bacon, than go to Heaven with Paley and Malthus" (Shelley, *Poetical* 207).

4. Working within a similarly satirical frame, canto XXXVIII of Byron's *Don Juan* (1826) laments how Malthus "turn[s] marriage into arithmetic"—yet, Don Juan continues:

> Had Adeline read Malthus? I can't tell;
> I wish she had: his book's the eleventh commandment,
> Which says, 'Thou shalt not marry,' unless *well*:
> This he (as far as I can understand) meant. (Byron, *Poetical Works* 836)

Byron's interest in Malthus had been piqued by a personal meeting in 1813 (Beaty 19) and, as we shall see, suggests a complicated relationship to the controversial theorist's claims. Perhaps in keeping with Anne Mellor's assessment of Byron as the master of romantic irony (*Gender* 31), Don Juan's awkwardly bracketed disavowal can be read as reflecting modest doubts that the "Malthus" demonized by literary figures like Percy Shelley in fact coincides with the *Essay*'s contents.

5. See Rajan and Wright's "Introduction" to *Romanticism, History and the Possibilities of Genre: Re-forming Literature 1789–1837*; Poovey. In terms of exceptions to this oversight, McLane reads *Frankenstein* through the lens of the Godwin-Malthus controversy as "a parable of [Godwinian] pedagogic failure" (84), while Collings argues that *Frankenstein*'s implied engagement with Malthus's 1798 *Essay* presents "a radical critique . . . showing that his [Malthus's] demographic demystification of the subject is as disastrous as her father's earlier, utopian mystification had been" (*Monstrous* 196). Although Anne McWhir includes a brief excerpt from the *Essay* in Appendix D of her Broadview edition of *The Last Man* (398–399), the scope and function of Malthusian ideas in Shelley's fourth novel have yet to receive sustained consideration. More recently, see Emily Steinlight's *Populating the Novel: Literary Form and the Politics of Surplus Life* (2018), especially chapter 2.

6. Such ephebiphobic impressions persisted long after the rebellion. As Randel notes, conservatives regularly beheld Ireland in the guise of a gigantic monster unleashed upon the British people (1843); as late as 1882, John Tenniel's "The Irish Frankenstein" depicted Ireland as an enormous knife-wielding beast. Yet Tenniel's tiny caption betrays a Shelleyan recognition of British responsibility for its wayward Irish child: "The baneful and blood-stained Monster *** yet was it not my Master to the very extent that it was my Creature? ***."

7. G.R. Thompson's introduction to *Gothic Imagination: Essays in Dark Romanticism* summarizes the subgenre like this: "Fallen man's inability fully to comprehend haunting reminders of another, supernatural realm that yet seemed not to exist, the constant perplexity of inexplicable and vastly metaphysical phenomena, a propensity for seemingly perverse or evil moral choices that had no firm or fixed measure or rule, and a sense of nameless guilt combined with a suspicion the external world was a delusive projection of the mind—these were major elements in the vision of man the Dark Romantics opposed to the mainstream of Romantic thought" (6).

8. See Wallace, "Keats's Frailty: The Body and Biography"; also Pyle, " 'Frail Spells': Shelley and the Ironies of Exile."

9. See Bailin and Kennedy for more on Victorian illness writing. For an assessment of Martineau's work from a disability studies perspective, see Frawley and Deegan.

Chapter 3

1. As De Quincey observed, "In short, up to 1820, the name of Wordsworth was trampled under foot; from 1820 to 1830 it was militant; from 1830 to 1835 it has been triumphant" ("Sketches" 543). Stephen Gill has explained how the last twenty-five years of Wordsworth's life saw his public reputation soar as his creative powers diminished; certain fellow poets, by contrast, had identified this decline years earlier, as Shelley's parodies and palinodes, or Byron's gleeful monikers ("Wordswords," "Turdsworth") attest.

2. This habit is consistent with Michel Foucault's observation in his essay "What is an Author?" which points out modern literary criticism's reluctance to view the author as anything but "the principle of a certain unity of writing—all differences [in a series of texts] having to be resolved, at least in part, by the principles of evolution, maturation, or influence" (111).

3. William A. Cohen and Ryan Johnson have distinguished between the economic figuration of waste as excess or superabundance and the comparably disgusting (although "conceivably productive" [x]) waste defined by threatening, toxic alterity: that is, the fearful and polluting "repositories of decay and death, feces and corpses" closely affiliated with the condemnatory *filth* (ix). Certainly there exist Victorian novels in which agedness is vehemently expressed as diseased excess and untouchable waste. In such cases, disgust is a prevalent and particularly dangerous affective response to the aged body, manifest in acts of psychological and physical abuse, even murder. In *Geronticide: Killing the Elderly* (2001), Mike Brogden states that the affective language of contamination renders the older person a mere "waste commodity" (21), forcibly distanced from personhood and thus "fit for disposal as detritus" (21). More than a century earlier, in *The Expression of the Emotions in Man and Animals* (1871), Charles Darwin summarized succinctly the affective dynamics of elder abuse evinced in Dickens and Trollope: "A person who is scorned is treated like dirt" (256).

4. See Charise (2012) for more discussion of Trollope's disgusted visions of old age in his late novel *The Fixed Period*.

5. In addition to Shuttleworth's essential 1986 volume, see Davis, Paxton, and Rylance for discussions of Eliot's engagement with Lewesian psychology.

6. I am grateful to Suzanne Raitt for her permission to cite her conference paper, "Waste and Repair in Wilde's *Dorian Gray*," delivered at the Interdisciplinary Nineteenth-Century Studies Conference (INCS) in 2011.

7. See also Zwierlein for a recent examination of Lewes's physiological writings on aging.

8. This dual nature of the spendthrift life is precisely at stake in Wilde's *The Picture of Dorian Gray*, for example, in which Dorian enjoys the splendid returns of his luscious experiences by mysteriously walling off his bodily life from the portrait that wastes away in the attic. In fact, Dorian's physiological squandering might be read as the other face of miserdom; the unnaturally youthened hedonist

and the parsimonious miser each hoard what protects against total dissipation, be it economic capital or the abstracted capital of youth itself.

9. As opposed to eighteenth-century metaphors of the machine, M.H. Abrams lucidly observes, the organicist model associated with Kant emphasized principles of wholeness (wherein individual parts are subordinated to the priority of the whole), growth (the whole is of an extensive and extending nature), assimilation (the conversion of diversity into unity with the whole), internality (the possession of spontaneous or *ab intra* energy for such growth), and interdependence (internally, between parts, but also between parts and whole). See *The Mirror and the Lamp*, especially chapters 7 and 8.

10. See Gullette's *Declining to Decline*. To name a Victorian exemplar of such imagery, the outset of chapter 31 in Thomas Hardy's *The Mayor of Casterbridge* contains a strong description of the protagonist Henchard's downward momentum on the downward slope of life: "Small as the police-court incident had been in itself, it formed the edge or turn in the incline of Henchard's fortunes. On that day—almost at that minute—he passed the ridge of prosperity and honour, and began to descend rapidly on the other side. It was strange how soon he sank in esteem. Socially he had received a startling fillip downwards; and, having already lost commercial buoyancy from rash transactions, the velocity of his descent in both aspects became accelerated every hour."

11. In *Topographies*, literary critic J. Hillis Miller investigates the significance of topographical language to nineteenth- and twentieth-century literature and philosophy, with particular attention to the way in which localizing terms and descriptions link features of landscape and their mapping to personification. Topography, he suggests, "originally meant the creation of a metaphorical equivalent in words of a landscape. Then, by another transfer, it came to mean representation of a landscape according to the conventional signs of some system of mapping" (3–4). Etymologically, topography combines the Greek word for "place" (τόπος, *topos*) with *gráphein* (γράφειν, to write) to indicate the writing, description, or naming of a landscape—imaginary or real—as place. In literature, the effects of this transfer are at once obvious and subtle: topography, in its "virtual writing" of the conventional signs of a terrain, alternates between connotations of "creating" and "revealing" those features, that region, this character, which is mapped (4). In the language of philosophy and criticism, topographical terminology like "method" (indicative of "the way"), "ground," or "field" translate their original referents into a conceptual vocabulary. In turn, such terminology provides "transparent illustrative metaphors, handy ways of thinking" (7).

12. See John McPhee's *Basin and Range* for an early usage of this phrase.

13. For key references to the "stages" model of aging and the broader dramatic conceptual framework that has shaped Western visions of the life-course, see Cole; also Marshall and Lipscomb.

14. Laura Diachun, MD. Personal interview. Apr. 2013.

15. Hence Lewes's profound skepticism that there exists any meaningful distinction between inorganic and organic elements: "No one has ever found that the elements of organic bodies differed, when separated, from those same elements in inorganic bodies. . . . There can be no such thing as matter essentially dead; there can be no such thing as matter essentially living. That which to-day we class as dead, will to-morrow be classed as living, and that which is living to-day will be dead to-morrow" (2:348).

16. It is significant that *The Physiology of Common Life* begins by critiquing the non-specificity of Kant's organicist definition of a living organism, asserting that if life is understood "as that in which each part is at once means and end," then such conditions "may be said with equal truth of fermentation" (2:355). As Sally Shuttleworth has shown, Lewes, Herbert Spencer, and Eliot were among the many Victorian intellectuals who saw physiological organization as consistent with larger psychological and social models. Shuttleworth's primary focus, however, is on the relationship of these writers' evolving organicism and its implications for the unconscious life of the mind (a topic that, as we know well, has far-reaching implications for Eliot's complex psychological portraits throughout her oeuvre). I reorient this established intellectual nexus to focus on the literary imagination of waste and repair, an idea, as Eliot and other novelists sensed, that carries with it implications for social as well as physiological life.

17. In *The Victorians and Old Age*, Karen Chase confirms the common impression generated by the Victorian period, namely, that it was an epoch often, even obsessively, associated with older age. Chase's astute analysis focuses on "nodal moments of intersection between narrative and cultural experience," primarily the ways in which old age was both reflected and formulated through fiction, journalism, the arts, and social policy (1). However, compared to Chase's comprehensive and persuasive discussion of the intersection of health policy and literary representations of aging, the productive porosity of medical and scientific thinking around aging remains somewhat indistinct. I am tempted to conclude that this why George Eliot is mentioned only three times in passing in this otherwise wide-ranging study of Victorian aging. By contrast, the novels of Charles Dickens—an author whom Lewes once found "mystifyingly indifferent" to matters of science—constitute the backbone of Chase's study (see Winyard and Fernaux).

18. Representative examples include Barbara Hardy's famous inference that Casaubon's association with dryness indicates his impotence (significantly, aridity has long been associated with the aging process by writers as historically and epistemologically divergent as Aristotle, Cicero, and Montaigne); or Heath's "Casaubon is a poor match for his young wife, made more so by his obliviousness to the significance of their twenty-seven year age difference, the fact that he is a generation older than his bride" (*Aging By the Book* 57); or that "Casaubon's decision to marry a 'blooming young lady' . . . is criticized through its devastating failure" (King 157).

19. This reference is too ubiquitous to be cited comprehensively here. To name a few representative examples: Jeff Nunokawa uses it in the title of his article, "The Miser's Two Bodies"; in *Unsettled Accounts: Money and Narrative in the Novels of George Gissing*, Simon J. James refers to "Eliot's miser Silas Marner" (11); and even Wikipedia's entry for "Miser" lists Marner as a classic example of the type (en.wikipedia.org/wiki/Miser).

20. See, for example, Capuano's *Changing Hands: Industry, Evolution, and the Reconfiguration of the Victorian Body* (2015) and Gilbert's article "The Will to Touch: David Copperfield's Hand" (2014).

21. Perhaps such trivialities are more at home in our own time than we realize. Social isolation is now understood as a risk factor for both physical and mental health problems in older people; a study recently published in the *American Journal of Geriatric Psychiatry* sought to evaluate whether an intergenerational volunteering program could enhance the quality of life of older persons with mild-to-moderate dementia. One of the interventions this study measured was physical contact between younger and older people—a finding that Eliot understood more than a century and a half ago. See George and Singer, "Intergenerational Volunteering and Quality of Life for Persons With Mild to Moderate Dementia."

22. As Robbins has noted, Brooke's mention of Peru is drawn from Johnson's 1749 "Vanity of Human Wishes" ("Let Observation, with extensive view, / Survey mankind from China to Peru" [1–2]). In the context of this short paragraph, the vanity of human wishes aligns with the narrator's chiding of youthful myopia. That age offers a lengthened view of experience is hardly an innovative position, and yet, the hints of geological catastrophism evident here refresh Eliot's recapitulation of this idea. The human time of youth is distinct from that of older age for whom "each shock" of the present (the literal and figurative "earthquakes") possesses a beginning, a middle, and an end, to repeat again within and beyond the purview of one's own lifespan.

Chapter 4

1. This passage, like much of Nordau's text, is rendered almost verbatim in the English translation of 1895. For example: "[G]reisenhaft ihr Lallen [babbling], Faseln [prating], Irrereden [ravings], und Fadenverlieren [lost threads]" (see *Entartung* 550–551). The Latinates included in the English translation effect a tone that closely matches Nordau's overwrought rhetoric and indexing in the original German.

2. Like Charles Darwin, who distinguished the endurance of biological species from the comparative instability of varieties ("incipient species"), Nordau's apprehension of new forms in *Degeneration* finds its expression in metaphors of youth and longevity (Darwin, *Origin* 44). However, Nordau's taxonomic vision of emergent varieties lacks Darwin's insistence that "species" is merely a convenient

term and not the name of an actual entity; see Darwin's *On The Origin of Species* (1859), especially chapter 2, "Variation Under Nature."

3. Sociologist of aging Stephen Katz notes, "In a society in which more women than men are diagnosed with AD [Alzheimer's dementia], in which more women than men are treated for mild cognitive impairment (MCI), and in which women are living longer than men, the gender implications for hypercognitive standards also complicate how the biosocial structuring of bodily life is impacting gender relations"; see Katz's "Embodied" (n.p.).

4. See Miller's *Topographies*. For a gloss of this work's key definitions and claims as they are relevant to my argument, see note 11 to chapter 3 above.

5. Kristeva's ideas have given rise to several important studies that consider the ways in which temporality can express queer subjectivities (see Marcus, Sedgwick, and Port, for example).

6. The *OED* lists a number of definitions that express the counterfeit's intrinsic ambiguity: "fashioned, made after a pattern" "imitation," "disguised," "not genuine," "represented by a picture or image," "pretended." In addition to literary texts motivated by these themes (for example, André Gide's 1925 novel *Les Faux-Monnayeurs* [*The Counterfeiters*, English trans. 1927]), the counterfeit speaks to the connections that exist between the self and commodity culture. As Scott Carpenter points out, there exists an unavoidable "lexical slippage" between the related terms and terminology of falsity, a slippage that reproduces exactly the conceptual blurring of boundaries and distinctions generated by deceptive things themselves (2). The counterfeit therefore refers not only to the unauthorized publication of texts, but also to a literary theme, political imagery, and even "a model and metaphor for literary production" (3). Rather than eluding or effacing our critical understanding of these phenomena, Carpenter argues that the inescapably fluid relationship between counterfeit, fraudulence, and authenticity in fact gets at the very truth of these concepts.

7. Charcot is best known as Sigmund Freud's mentor at the Salpêtrière Hospital in Paris and for his medical investigation (and, as some would argue, choreography) of the condition once known as hysteria. Decades before, Charcot was internationally recognized for his pioneering investigations into the etiology of illnesses in older people, and elderly women in particular (the so-called "senile diseases"). Little scholarship has addressed the intriguing fact that the medical constructs of hysteria and senility were born in the same hospital and under Charcot's watch; but see Katz's *Disciplining*, especially chapter 3, "Textual Formations and the Science of Old Age."

8. By making this claim I do not mean to suggest that all or even most *fin de siècle* representations of the non-conventional female subject portrayed her as nonreproductive or asexual. For example, Grant Allen's *The Woman Who Did* (1895) or Sarah Grand's *The Heavenly Twins* (1893) each explore the complexities of women's sexual relationships and childbirth both inside and outside of the constraints of wedlock.

9. Orwell laments the difficulty had in procuring copies of Gissing's novels, perhaps most of all because he was "ready to maintain that England has produced very few better novelists" (429). *New Grub Street*, he writes, only exists in "soupstained copies borrowed from public lending libraries," while *The Odd Women* "is about as thoroughly out of print as a book can be" (429). Since that time, Gissing's star has risen impressively: new annotated scholarly editions of his major and comparatively minor works are widely available, as are biographies (Pierre Coustillas's three-volume *Life of George Gissing* was published in 2012), international conferences, critical articles, and increased visibility of Gissing's works on undergraduate syllabi.

10. In her fundamental book *Powers of Horror: An Essay on Abjection* (1980), Julia Kristeva defines the "abject" not so much as the disgusting or repellant thing itself, but as that which threatens identity by undermining corporeal stability. "It is thus not lack of cleanliness or health that causes abjection," Kristeva writes, "but what disturbs identity, system, order. What does not respect borders, positions, rules. The in-between, the ambiguous, the composite" (4).

11. Everard's and Gissing's references to "old" ways evoke an intertextual resonance with the seventeenth-century tragicomedy *The Old Law, or A New Way to Please You* (1656), written by Thomas Middleton, William Rowley, and Philip Massinger. A partial source for Anthony Trollope's speculative fiction satire *The Fixed Period* (1881) discussed in chapter 5, *The Old Law* is the staging of a dystopian society where elderly men (at the age of eighty) and women (at the age of sixty) are put to death by being thrown from a cliff into the sea: a fate not unlike Gloucester's attempted suicide in Shakespeare's earlier tragedy *King Lear*.

12. Daniel Hack has recently argued that Tennyson's "The Charge of the Light Brigade" was de- and re-contextualized in the context of African-American debates over antislavery violence. As he argues, "the recovery of this tradition promises to produce a more capacious understanding of the cultural work Tennyson's warhorse of a poem has been called upon to perform" (201). My discussion of Tennyson reads "The Charge of the Light Brigade" in a similar vein, arguing that Kipling's uptake of Tennyson's subjects, like Gissing's portrayal of surplus women, makes visible literary and social strategies of obscuring the human lives deemed superfluous by temporal conventions.

13. My research suggests that this phrase was widely used at the end of the nineteenth century but its source remains mysterious and possibly apocryphal. In 1887 Nellie Maclagan asks, "Who is the author of this much-cited phrase?" in *Notes and Queries* (189), but her question remains unanswered. Among other instances, in an October 1885 lecture entitled "Culture and Science" published in *Macmillan's Magazine* (1886), professor of classics Edward Adolf (E.A.) Sonnenschein states that "the 'so-called nineteenth century,' as an indignant and sarcastic lecturer is said to have called it, is marked by a powerful re-action against the tradition of an exclusive classical education" (9); the *OED* further notes that in an 1888 editorial in *The Woman's World* entitled "Literary and Other Notes," Oscar Wilde writes,

"Nothing is more interesting than to watch the change and development of the art of novel-writing in this nineteenth century—'this so-called nineteenth century,' as an impassioned young orator once termed it, after a contemptuous diatribe against the evils of modern civilization" (134)." As Wilde's usage illustrates, the phrase is often cited in literary and journalistic texts from the mid-1880s onward, often alongside references to a (variously) "impassioned" "orator," "lecturer," or "reverend" (often "young"), who was delivering a speech about the evils or false claims of "modern civilization" (sometimes "science." The earliest reference I can locate occurs in an 1877 volume of the *Sunday Magazine* in an article on Roger Bacon, and gives the impression that the phrase is somewhat recent.

14. Sandra Gilbert and Susan Gubar describe Ayesha as "neither an angel or a monster. Rather, *She-who-must-be-obeyed* was an odd blend of the two types—an angelically chaste woman with monstrous powers, a monstrously passionate woman with angelic charms. Just as importantly, however, She was in certain ways an entirely New Woman: the all-knowing, all-powerful ruler of a matriarchal society" (*No Man's Land* 6).

15. More recently, Kay Heath has discussed the manifold forms of Victorian "age anxiety" that regularly invoke Woodward's notion of youth-as-masquerade. Such examples of anti-aging culture regularly took the shape of advertisements for soap, pills, balms, and lotions that "project[ed] fears of national decline onto the commercialized, midlife body" (*Aging* 173). Heath even cites Nordau's *Degeneration* as an example of the late-century habit of associating urbanizing forces of modern life with societal ills and cultural decline.

16. For another treatment of literary "senility," see Chase's "Senile Sexuality."

Chapter 5

1. See W. L. Collins's note in *Blackwood's* cited in Smalley, *Anthony Trollope*, 492. Sam Silverman's essay "Trollope's The Fixed Period: A Nineteenth-Century Novel Revisited" gives a comprehensive sense of Trollope's compounding depression at the time of writing this novel.

Works Cited

Abrams. M.H. *The Mirror and the Lamp: Romantic Theory and the Critical Tradition.* Oxford UP, 1971.
Alighieri, Dante. "Inferno." *The Norton Anthology of World Masterpieces*, translated by Allen Mandelbaum, 7th ed., vol. 1., Norton, 1999, pp. 1303–1428.
Allen, Grant. "Plain Words on the Woman Question." *Fortnightly Review* 46 (1889), pp. 448–458.
Antonovsky, Aaron. "Social Class, Life Expectancy and Overall Mortality." *The Milbank Memorial Fund Quarterly* 45.1 (1967), pp. 31–73.
Aristotle. *On Longevity and Shortness of Life.* Translated by G.R.T. Ross, Alex Catalogue, n.d.
Armstrong, Tim. *Modernism, Technology, and the Body: A Cultural Study.* Cambridge UP, 1998.
Arnold, Matthew. "Growing Old." *Victorian and Edwardian Poets: Tennyson to Yeats*, Viking Press, 1965, pp. 210–211.
Aschoff, Jurgen. "Bicentennial Anniversary of Christoph Wilhelm Hufeland's Die Kunst als menschliche Leben zu verlängern (The Art of Prolonging Human Life)." *Journal of Biological Rhythms* 13.1 (1998), pp. 4–8.
Bailin, Mariam. *The Sickroom in Victorian Fiction: The Art of Being Ill.* Cambridge UP, 1994.
Bakhtin, Mikhail. *The Dialogic Imagination: Four Essays.* Edited by Michael Holquist, translated by Caryl Emerson and Michael Holquist, U of Texas P, 1981.
Balkun, Mary McAleer. *The American Counterfeit: Authenticity and Identity in American Literature and Culture.* U of Alabama P, 2006.
Ballenger, Jesse. *Self, Senility, and Alzheimer's Disease in Modern America: A History.* Johns Hopkins UP, 2006.
Baltes, Paul B., and Jacqui Smith. "New Frontiers in the Future of Aging: From Successful Aging of the Young Old to the Dilemmas of the Fourth Age." *Gerontology* 49.2 (2003), pp. 123–135.
Beaty, Frederick L. "Byron on Malthus and the Population Problem." *Keats-Shelley Journal* 18 (1969), pp. 17–26.

Beddoes, Thomas. *Hygëia: or Essays Moral and Medical on the Causes Affecting the Personal State of One Middling and Affluent Classes*. J. Mills, 1802. 3 vols.
Beer, Gillian. *Darwin's Plots*, 3rd edition, Cambridge UP, 2009.
Bender, John. "Enlightenment Fiction and the Scientific Hypothesis." *Representations* 61 (1998), pp. 6–28.
Benjamin, Walter. *Origin of the German Trauerspiel*. Translated by Howard Eiland, Harvard UP, 2019.
———. "The Work of Art in the Age of Mechanical Reproduction." *Illuminations*, edited by Hannah Arendt, translated by Harry Zohn, Schocken Books, 1969.
Berlin, Isaiah. *The Roots of Romanticism*. Edited by Henry Hardy, Princeton UP, 1999.
Bewell, Alan. *Romanticism and Colonial Disease*. Johns Hopkins UP, 1999.
———. *Wordsworth and the Enlightenment: Nature, Man, and Society in the Experimental Poetry*. Yale UP, 1989.
The Bible. Authorized King James Version [*The Holy Bible, Conteyning the Old Testament, and the New: Newly Translated out of the Originall tongues: & with the former Translations diligently compared and reuised by his Maiesties speciall Comandement. Appointed to be read in Churches*]. London: Robert Barker, 1611.
Black, Clementina. "The Odd Women." *Illustrated London News* 155 (5 Aug. 1893).
Blake, William. *Songs of Innocence and of Experience*. Oxford UP, 1970.
Blakemore, Steven. "Burke and the Fall of Language." *Edmund Burke: Appraisals and Applications*, edited by Daniel Ritchie, Transaction, 1990.
Bloom, Harold. *The Anxiety of Influence: A Theory of Poetry*. Oxford UP, 1973.
Bonar, J. "The Centenary of Malthus." *The Economic Journal* 8.30 (1898), pp. 206–208.
Brewer, William D. *The Mental Anatomies of William Godwin and Mary Shelley*. Fairleigh-Dickinson UP, 2001.
Brogden, Mike. *Geronticide: Killing the Elderly*. Jessica Kingsley, 2001.
Browning, Robert. "An Essay on Shelley." *The Broadview Anthology of Victorian Poetry and Poetic Theory, Concise Edition*, edited by Thomas J. Collins and Vivienne J. Rundle, Broadview, 2000.
———. "Rabbi Ben Ezra." *The Poems and Plays of Robert Browning*. Modern Library, 1934, p. 291.
Burke, Edmund. *The Writings and Speeches of Edmund Burke: Volume I: The Early Writings*. Edited by T.O. McLoughlin and James T. Boulton, Oxford UP, 1997.
Byron, George Gordon. *The Works of Lord Byron: Letters and Journals*. Edited by Rowland E. Prothero, Charles Scribner's Sons, 1901.
———. *The Poetical Works of Byron*. Oxford UP, n.d.
Capuano, Peter J. *Changing Hands: Industry, Evolution, and the Reconfiguration of the Victorian Body*. U of Michigan P, 2015.
Carlyle, Thomas. *Critical and Miscellaneous Essays, Volume 2*. Boston: Munroe, 1839.
Carpenter, Scott. *Aesthetics of Fraudulence in Nineteenth-Century France: Frauds, Hoaxes, and Counterfeits*. Ashgate, 2009.

Carroll, Lewis. *The Annotated Alice: The Definitive Edition*. Edited by Martin Gardner, W.W. Norton, 1999.
Chandler, Anne. "Romanticizing Adolescence: Godwin's St. Leon and the Matter of Rousseau." *Studies for Romanticism* 41.3 (2002), pp. 399–414.
Chandler, James. *England in 1819: The Politics of Literary Culture and the Case of Romantic Historicism*. U of Chicago P, 1998.
"Character Note: The New Woman." *Cornhill* 136 (1894), pp. 365–368.
Charcot, Jean-Martin. *Clinical Lectures of Senile and Chronic Diseases*. Arno, 1979.
Charise, Andrea. "The Future is Certain: Manifesting Age, Culture, Humanities." *Age, Culture, Humanities: An Interdisciplinary Journal* 1 (2014), pp. 11–16.
———. "G.H. Lewes and the Impossible Classification of Organic Life." *Victorian Studies* 57.3 (2015), pp. 377–386.
———. " 'Let the Reader Think of the Burden': Old Age and the Crisis of Capacity." *Occasion: Interdisciplinary Studies in the Humanities* 4 (2012), pp. 1–16.
———. "Romanticism Against Youth." *Essays in Romanticism* 20.1 (2013), pp. 83–100.
———. " 'The Tyranny of Age': Godwin's *St. Leon* and the Nineteenth-Century Longevity Narrative." *English Literary History* 79.4 (2012), pp. 905–933.
Chase, Karen. *The Victorians and Old Age*. Oxford UP, 2009.
———. "The Coming of Age II." *Journal of Victorian Culture* 16.1 (2011), pp. 128–132.
———. "Senile Sexuality." *Interdisciplinary Perspectives on Ageing in Nineteenth-Century Culture*, edited by Katharina Boehm, Anna Farkas, and Anne Zwierlein, Routledge, 2013, pp. 132–146.
Cicero, Marcus Tullius. *De Senectute*. Translate by William Armistead Falconer, Loeb Classical Library, 2001.
Cohen, William A. *Embodied: Victorian Literature and the Senses*. U of Minnesota P, 2009.
Cohen, William A., and Ryan Johnson. *Filth: Dirt, Disgust, and Modern Life*. U of Minnesota P, 2005.
Cole, Thomas R. *The Journey of Life: A Cultural History of Aging in America*. Cambridge UP, 1992.
Colella, Silvana. "Intimations of Mortality: The Malthusian Plot in Early Nineteenth-Century Popular Fiction." *Nineteenth-Century Contexts* 24.1 (2002), pp. 17–32.
Coleridge, Samuel Taylor. *The Major Works*. Oxford UP, 2008.
———. *Specimens of the Table Talk of the Late Samuel Taylor Coleridge, Volume 2*. London: John Murray, 1835.
Collings, David. "Covenant in Hyperbole: The Disruption of Tradition in 'Michael.' " *Studies in Romanticism* 32.4 (1993), pp. 551–576.
———. *Monstrous Society: Reciprocity, Discipline, and the Political Uncanny at the End of Early Modern England*. Bucknell UP, 2009.

———. "The Romance of the Impossible: William Godwin in the Empty Place of Reason." *English Literary History* 70.3 (2003), pp. 847–874.
Cook, Susan E. "Envisioning Reform in Gissing's *The Nether World*." *English Literature in Transition, 1880–1920* 52.4 (2009), pp. 458–475.
Corkhill, Alan. "Charlatanism in Goethe's *Faust I* and Tieck's *William Lovell*." *Forum for Modern Language Studies* 42.1 (2005), pp. 80–92.
Cottingham, John. "Introduction." *The Cambridge Companion to Descartes*. Cambridge UP, 1992.
Crichton-Browne, James. "The Annual Oration on Sex in Education." *British Medical Journal* 1637 (7 May 1892), pp. 949–954.
———. *The Prevention of Senility, and A Sanitary Outlook*. Macmillan and Co., 1905.
Cruikshank, Margaret. *Learning to Be Old: Gender, Culture, and Aging*. 2nd ed., Rowman and Littlefield, 2009.
Crump, Justine. "Gambling, History, and Godwin's *St. Leon*." *European Romantic Review* 11 (2009), pp. 393–407.
Dames, Nicholas. *The Physiology of the Novel: Reading, Neural Science, and the Form of the Victorian Novel*. Oxford UP, 2007.
———. "Untimely Contextualizations." *Journal of Victorian Culture* 16.1 (2011), pp. 113–117.
Darwin, Charles. *The Descent of Man and Selection in Relation to Sex*. New York: D. Appleton and Company, 1896.
———. *The Expression of the Emotions in Man and Animals*. New York: D. Appleton and Company, 1886.
———. *On the Origin of Species*. Edited by Gillian Beer, Oxford UP, 1998.
Darwin, Erasmus. *The Botanic Garden, A Poem, in Two Parts; Containing The Economy of Vegetation and The Loves of the Plants*. London: J. Johnson, 1799.
———. *The Temple of Nature; Or, The Origin of Society: A Poem with Philosophical Notes*. Echo, 2009.
———. *Zoonomia; Or, The Laws of Organic Life. In Four Volumes*. London: J. Johnson, 1801.
Davis, Michael. *George Eliot and Nineteenth-Century Psychology: Exploring the Unmapped Country*. Ashgate, 2006.
Day, George E. *A Practical Treatise on the Domestic Management and Most Important Diseases of Advanced Life*. Philadelphia: Lea and Blanchard, 1849.
De Almeida, Hermione. *Romantic Medicine and John Keats*. Oxford UP, 1991.
de Beauvoir, Simone. *The Coming of Age [La Vieillesse]*. Translated by Patrick O'Brian, Putnam, 1972.
Deegan, Mary Jo. "Making Lemonade: Harriet Martineau on Being Deaf." *Harriet Martineau: Theoretical and Methodological Perspectives*, edited by Michael R. Hill and Susan Hoecker-Drysdale, Routledge, 2001.
De Quincey, Thomas. *Collected Writings*. Edited by David Masson, London: A. & C. Black, 1896–97.

———. *Confessions of an English Opium-Eater and Other Writings*. Oxford UP, 1998.
———. *Recollections of the Lake Poets*. Edited by Edward Sackville-West, Lehmann, 1948.
———. "Sketches of Life and Manners: From the Autobiography of an Opium Eater. Oxford." *Tait's Edinburgh Magazine* 2 (1835), pp. 541–550.
Descartes, Rene. *Discours de la Méthode & Essais. Oeuvres de Descartes*, edited by Charles Adam and Paul Tannery, Léopold Cerf, 1902.
———. "The Passions of the Soul." *The Philosophical Writings of Rene Descartes*, edited by John Cottingham, Robert Stoothoff, and Dugald Murdoch, vol. 1, Cambridge UP, 1984.
Dickens, Charles. *A Christmas Carol*. Broadview, 2003.
———. *Little Dorrit*. New York: Sheldon and Co., 1863.
———. *Our Mutual Friend*. Random House, 2002.
Donne, John. *Paradoxes and Problems*. Nonesuch Press, 1923.
Du Halde, Jean-Baptiste. *A Description of the Empire of China and Chinese-Tartary, Together with the Kingdoms of Korea, and Tibet*. London: T. Gardner, 1744.
Eagleton, Terry. *The Ideology of the Aesthetic*. Blackwell, 1990.
Edelman, Lee. *No Future: Queer Theory and the Death Drive*. Duke UP, 2005.
Eliot, George. *Daniel Deronda*. Wordsworth Editions, 1996.
———. *Essays*. Edited by Thomas Pinney, Routledge, 1963.
———. *Life And Letters: The Works of George Eliot*. Kessinger, 2004.
———. *Middlemarch: A Study of Provincial Life*. Pan, 1973.
———. *Scenes of Clerical Life*. Oxford UP, 2000.
———. *Silas Marner: The Weaver of Raveloe*. Wordsworth Editions, 1999.
Ette, Ottmar. "Literature as Knowledge for Living, Literary Studies as Science for Living." Translated by Vera M. Kutzinski, *PMLA* 125.4 (2010), pp. 977–993.
Ferguson, Frances. *Solitude and the Sublime: Romanticism and the Aesthetics of Individuation*. Routledge, 1992.
Ferris, Ina. *The Romantic National Tale and the Question of Ireland*. Cambridge UP, 2002.
Fisch, Audrey A. "Plaguing Politics: AIDS, Deconstruction, and The Last Man." *The Other Mary Shelley: Beyond Frankenstein*, edited by Audrey A. Fisch, Anne Kostelanetz Mellor, and Esther H. Schor, Oxford UP, 1993.
Fisch, Audrey A., Anne Kostelanetz Mellor, and Esther H. Schor, eds. *The Other Mary Shelley: Beyond Frankenstein*. Oxford UP, 1993.
Fliegelman, Jay. *Prodigals and Pilgrims: The American Revolution Against Patriarchal Authority, 1750–1800*. Cambridge UP, 1982.
Flourens, Pierre. *De la longévité humaine et de la quantité de vie sur le globe [On Human Longevity, and the Amount of Life Upon the Globe]*. Paris: Garnier Frères, 1855.

Flynn, Carol Houlihan. "Running Out of Matter: The Body Exercised in Eighteenth-Century Fiction." *The Languages of Psyche: Mind and Body in Enlightenment Thought*, edited by G. S. Rousseau, U of California P, 1990, pp. 147–185.

Ford, Jennifer. *Coleridge on Dreaming: Romanticism, Dreams and the Medical Imagination*. Cambridge UP, 1998.

Foucault, Michel. *The Birth of the Clinic: An Archaeology of Medical Perception*. Translated by Alan Sheridan, Routledge, 2003.

———. *Discipline and Punish: The Birth of the Prison*. Translated by Alan Sheridan, Random House, 1995.

———. *The History of Sexuality: Volume 1: An Introduction*. Translated by Robert Hurley, Random House, 1978.

———. "What is an Author?" *The Foucault Reader*, edited by Paul Rabinow, Pantheon, 1984.

Fox, Robert. "The Many Worlds of Thomas Beddoes." *Notes and Records of the Royal Society* 63.3 (2009), pp. 211–213.

Frawley, Maria. *Invalidism and Identity in Nineteenth-Century Britain*. U of Chicago P, 2004.

Froide, Amy M. *Never Married: Singlewomen in Early Modern England*. Oxford UP, 2005.

Fulford, Tim. "Apocalyptic Economics and Prophetic Politics: Radical and Romantic Responses to Malthus and Burke." *Studies in Romanticism* 40.3 (2001), pp. 345–368.

Gallagher, Catherine. *The Body Economic: Life, Death, and Sensation in Political Economy and the Victorian Novel*. Princeton UP, 2008.

———. "The Rise of Fictionality." *The Novel*. Edited by Franco Moretti, vol. 1, Princeton UP, 2006, pp. 336–363.

Gaskell, Elizabeth. *Cranford*. Edited by Elizabeth Langland. Broadview, 2010.

George, Daniel R., and Mendel E. Singer. "Intergenerational Volunteering and Quality of Life for Persons with Mild to Moderate Dementia: Results from a 5-Month Intervention Study in the United States." *American Journal of Geriatric Psychiatry* 19.4 (2011), pp. 392–396.

Gibbon, Edward. *The Decline and Fall of the Roman Empire*. London: Cadell, 1837.

Gilbert, Pamela K. "The Will to Touch: David Copperfield's Hand." *19: Interdisciplinary Studies in the Long Nineteenth Century* 19 (2014), pp. 1–15.

Gilbert, Sandra, and Susan Gubar. *No Man's Land: The Place of the Woman Writer in the Twentieth Century. Volume 2: Sexchanges*. Yale UP, 1989.

Gill, Stephen. *Wordsworth and the Victorians*. Clarendon, 1998.

Gissing, George. *The Odd Women*. Edited by Arlene Young, Broadview, 2002.

———. "The Place of Realism in Fiction." *Nineteenth-Century British Novelists on the Novel*, edited by George L. Barnett, Appleton-Century-Crofts, 1968, pp. 314–316.

"Godwin on Malthus." *The Edinburgh Review, or, Critical Journal* 35 (1821), pp. 362–377.

Godwin, William. *Caleb Williams*. Edited by Gary Handwerk and A.A. Markley, Broadview, 2000.

———. *Catalogue of the Curious Library of That Very Eminent and Distinguished Author, William Godwin, Esq.: To Which Are Added, the Very Interesting and Original Autograph Manuscripts of His Highly Esteemed Publications, Which Will Be Sold by Auction by Mr. Sotheby and Son on Friday, June 17th, 1836 and Following Day*. London: Sotheby and Son, 1836.

———. *The Diary of William Godwin*. Edited by Victoria Myers, David O'Shaughnessy, and Mark Philp, Oxford Digital Library, godwindiary.bodleian.ox.ac.uk, 2010.

———. *Enquiry Concerning Political Justice and its Influence on Modern Morals and Happiness*. Edited by F.E.L. Priestley, U of Toronto P, 1946. 3 vols.

———. *Of Population: An Enquiry Concerning the Power of Increase in the Numbers of Mankind, Being an Answer to Mr. Malthus's Essay on that Subject*. Longman, Hurst, Rees, Orme and Brown, 1820.

———. *St. Leon: A Tale of the Sixteenth Century*. Edited by William D. Brewer, Broadview, 2006.

———. *Thoughts Occasioned by The Perusal of Dr. Parr's Spital Sermon, Preached at Christ Church, April 15, 1800: Being a Reply to the Attacks of Dr. Parr, Mr. Mackintosh, the Author of an Essay on Population, and Others*. London: Taylor and Wilks, 1801.

Goldsmith, Steven. *Unbuilding Jerusalem: Apocalypse and Romantic Representation*. Cornell UP, 1993.

Goose, Nigel. "Poverty, Old Age and Gender in Nineteenth-Century England: The Case of Hertfordshire." *Continuity and Change* 20.3 (2005), pp. 351–384.

Graham, Kenneth W., ed. *William Godwin Reviewed: A Reception History 1783–1834*. AMS, 2001.

Grand, Sarah. *The Heavenly Twins*. Cassell, 1983.

Greg, William Rathbone. *Why Are Women Redundant?* London: Trubner, 1869.

Grosz, Elizabeth. "The Problem of Theory." *theory@buffalo* 5 (1999), pp. 2–16.

Gruman, Gerald J. *A History of Ideas about the Prolongation of Life*. Springer, 2003.

Gullette, Margaret Morganroth. *Aged by Culture*. U of Chicago P, 2004.

———. *Declining to Decline: Cultural Combat and the Politics of the Midlife*. UP of Virginia, 1997.

Hack, Daniel. "Wild Charges: The Afro-Haitian 'Charge of the Light Brigade'." *Victorian Studies* 54.2 (2012), pp. 199–225.

Haggard, H. Rider. *She*. Broadview, 2006.

Haight, Gordon S. *George Eliot: A Biography*. Penguin, 1985.

Halberstam, Jack. "What's That Smell? Queer Temporalities and Subcultural Lives." *The Scholar and Feminist Online* 2.1 (2003), n.p.

Hall, G. Stanley. *Senescence: The Last Half of Life*. Appleton and Company, 1922.

Handwerk, Gary. "History, Trauma, and the Limits of the Liberal Imagination: William Godwin's Historical Fiction." *Romanticism, History, and the Possibilities of Genre: Re-Forming Literature 1789–1837*, edited by Tilottama Rajan and Julia M. Wright, Cambridge UP, 1998, pp. 64–85.

Hardy, Barbara. *The Appropriate Form: An Essay on the Novel.* Athlone, 1964.

———. *George Eliot: A Critic's Biography.* Continuum, 2006.

Hardy, Thomas. *Jude the Obscure.* Broadview, 1999.

———. *The Mayor of Casterbridge: The Life and Death of a Man of Character.* Macmillan and Co., 1902.

———. *Poems of the Past and the Present.* Harper and Brothers, 1902.

Harvie, Jen. "Boom! Adversarial Ageism, Chrononormativity, and the Anthropocene." *Contemporary Theatre Review* 28.3 (2018), 332–344.

Hazlitt, William. "On the Old Age of Artists." *The Plain Speaker: The Key Essays*, edited by Duncan Wu and Tom Paulin, Wiley-Blackwell, 1998.

Heath, Kay. *Aging by the Book: The Emergence of Mid-Life in Victorian Britain.* SUNY P, 2009.

———. "In the Eye of the Beholder: Victorian Age Construction and the Specular Self." *Victorian Literature and Culture* 34.1 (2006), pp. 27–45.

Henry, Nancy. *The Cambridge Introduction to George Eliot.* Cambridge UP, 2008.

Heringman, Noah. *Romantic Rocks.* Cornell UP, 2004.

Higdon, David Leon. "George Eliot and the Art of the Epigraph." *Nineteenth-Century Fiction* 25.2 (1970), pp. 127–151.

Hill, Bridget. *Women Alone: Spinsters in England 1660–1850.* Yale UP, 2001.

"Historical Statistics on Population for the Country | Current rate: Percentage Aged over 65." *A Vision of Britain through Time.* U of Portsmouth. 15 Dec. 2018, www.visionofbritain.org.uk/unit/10042124/rate/AGE_65_up.

"Historical Statistics on Population for the Country | Rate: Rate of Population Change (% over previous 10 years)." *A Vision of Britain through Time.* U of Portsmouth. 15 Dec. 2018, www.visionofbritain.org.uk/unit/10061325/rate/POP_CH_10.

Hogle, Jerrold E. "The Gothic Ghost of the Counterfeit and the Progress of Abjection." *A New Companion to the Gothic*, edited by David Punter, Blackwell, 2012, pp. 496–509.

Hufeland, Christoph Wilhelm. *The Art of Prolonging Life.* Edited by Erasmus Wilson, Lindsay & Blakiston, 1867.

Hume, David. *An Enquiry Concerning Human Understanding: A Critical Edition.* Edited by Tom L. Beauchamp, Oxford UP, 2000.

———. *Selected Essays.* Oxford UP, 1993.

Hunt, Leigh. "Chevalier de Boufflers' 'Love and War.'" *The Poetical Works of Leigh Hunt*, London: Moxon, 1832, pp. 329–330.

James, Patricia. *Population Malthus: His Life and Times.* Routledge, 2006.

James, Simon J. *Unsettled Accounts: Money and Narrative in the Novels of George Gissing.* Anthem, 2003.

Jameson, Fredric. *Archaeologies of the Future: The Desire Called Utopia and Other Science Fictions*. Verso, 2005.
Johnson, Barbara. "The Last Man." *The Other Mary Shelley: Beyond Frankenstein*, edited by Audrey A. Fisch, Anne Kostelanetz Mellor, and Esther H. Schor, Oxford UP, 1993.
Johnson, Samuel. "The Vanity of Human Wishes." *A Collection of Poems in Four Volumes*. London: Printed by J. Hughs, for R. and J. Dodsley, 1755.
Joseph, Mark. "Have We Added Another Lost Generation?" *Huffington Post*, 11 June 2012, www.huffpost.com/entry/generation-z-summer-camps_b_1416380.
Katz, Stephen. "Embodied Memory: Ageing, Neuroculture, and the Genealogy of Mind." *Occasion: Interdisciplinary Studies in the Humanities* 4.31 (2012).
———. *Disciplining Old Age: The Formation of Gerontological Knowledge*. UP of Virginia, 1996.
Keats, John. *Complete Poems and Selected Letters of John Keats*. Random House, 2009.
Kelly, Gary. *The English Jacobin Novel, 1780–1805*. Clarendon, 1976.
Kennedy, Meghan. "The Victorian Novel and Medicine." *The Oxford Handbook of the Victorian Novel*, edited by Lisa Rodensky, Oxford UP, 2016, pp. 459–480.
King, Amy M. *Bloom: The Botanical Vernacular in the English Novel*. Oxford UP, 2003.
Kipling, Rudyard. "The Last of the Light Brigade." *Rudyard Kipling's Verse: Inclusive Edition 1885–1918*, Copp-Clark, 1919, pp. 228–230.
Knoepflmacher, U.C. *George Eliot's Early Novels: The Limits of Realism*. U of California P, 1968.
Kornbluh, Anna, and Benjamin Morgan. "Introduction: Presentism, Form, and the Future of History." *b2o: an online journal*, 4 Oct. 2016. www.boundary2.org/2016/10/anna-kornbluh-and-benjamin-morgan-introduction-presentism-form-and-the-future-of-history/.
Kranidis, Rita S. *The Victorian Spinster and Colonial Emigration: Contested Subjects*. St. Martin's Press, 1999.
Kristeva, Julia. *Powers of Horror: An Essay on Abjection*. Translated by Leon S. Roudiez, Columbia UP, 1982.
———. "Women's Time." Translated by Alice Jardine and Harry Blake. *The Kristeva Reader*. Edited by Toril Moi, Columbia UP, 1986, pp. 187–213.
Lamb, Charles. *Elia. The Last Essays of Elia. The Works of Charles Lamb*, vol. 3, edited by A.C. Armstrong, 1886.
Laslett, Peter. *A Fresh Map of Life: The Emergence of the Third Age*. Harvard UP, 1991.
Levere, Trevor H. *Poetry Realized in Nature: Samuel Taylor Coleridge and Early Nineteenth-Century Science*. Cambridge UP, 1981.
Lewes, George Henry. *The Physiology of Common Life*. Edinburgh: Blackwood, 1859. 2 vols.
"Long Life." *The Monthly Visitor, and Entertaining Pocket Companion*, vol. 7, London: H.D. Symonds, 1799, pp. 250–252.
Looser, Devoney. "Old Age and the End of Oblivion." *Journal of Victorian Culture* 16.1 (2011), pp. 132–137.

———. "'What the Devil a Woman Lives for After 30': The Late Careers of Late Eighteenth-Century Women Writers." *Journal of Aging and Identity* 4.1 (1999), pp. 3–11.

———. *Women Writers and Old Age in Great Britain, 1750–1850*. Johns Hopkins UP, 2008.

Lukács, György. *The Historical Novel*. Translated by Hannah and Stanley Mitchell, U of Nebraska P, 1983.

Lyell, Charles. *Principles of Geology: Being an Attempt to Explain the Former Changes of the Earth's Surface, by Reference to Causes Now in Operation*. London: John Murray, 1830. 2 vols.

Maclagan, Nellie. "This So-Called Nineteenth Century." *Notes and Queries*, 5 March 1887, p. 189.

Malthus, Thomas Robert. *An Essay on the Principle of Population and A Summary View of the Principle of Population*. Edited by Philip Appleman, Norton, 1976.

———. "Appendix, 1806." *An Essay on the Principle of Population*, edited by Donald Winch, Cambridge UP, 1992, pp. 333–365.

———. *The Travel Diaries of Thomas Robert Malthus*. Cambridge UP for the Royal Economic Society, 1966.

Mangum, Teresa. "Little Women: The Aging Female Character in Nineteenth-Century British Children's Literature." *Figuring Age: Women, Bodies, Generations*, edited by Kathleen Woodward, Indiana UP, 1999.

———. *Married, Middle-Brow, and Militant: Sarah Grand and the New Woman Novel*. U of Michigan P, 1998.

———. "Passages of Life: Growing Old." *A Companion to Victorian Literature and Culture*, edited by Herbert Tucker, Blackwell, 1999, pp. 97–109.

"Manifesto of the V21 Collective: Ten Theses." 2015. 15 Dec. 2018, v21collective.org/manifesto-of-the-v21-collective-ten-theses/.

Marche, Stephen. "The War Against Youth." *Esquire*, 26 Mar. 2012, www.esquire.com/news-politics/a13226/young-people-in-the-recession-0412/.

Marcus, Sharon. *Between Women: Friendship, Desire, and Marriage in Victorian England*. Princeton UP, 2007.

Marks, Patricia. *Bicycles, Bangs, and Bloomers: The New Woman in the Popular Press*. UP Kentucky, 1990.

Marshall, Leni. *Age Becomes US: Bodies and Gender in Time*. SUNY P, 2015.

Marshall, Leni, and Valerie Lipscomb, eds. *Staging Age: The Performance of Age in Theatre, Dance, and Film*. Palgrave Macmillan, 2010.

Marx, Steven. *Youth Against Age: Generational Strife in Renaissance Poetry*. Peter Lang, 1986.

Matz, Aaron. *Satire in an Age of Realism*. Cambridge UP, 2010.

May, Charles E. "Hardy's 'Darkling Thrush': The 'Nightingale' Grown Old." *Victorian Poetry* 11.1 (1973), pp. 62–65.

McDonagh, Josephine. "Infanticidal Mothers and Dead Babies: Women's Voices on Political Economy and Population." *Bells: Barcelona English Language and Literature Studies* 7 (1996), pp. 11–20.
McLane, Maureen N. *Romanticism and the Human Sciences: Poetry, Population, and the Discourse of the Species*. Cambridge UP, 2000.
McManners, John. *Death and the Enlightenment: Changing Attitudes to Death Among Christians and Unbelievers in Eighteenth-Century France*. Clarendon, 1981.
McPhee, John. *Basin and Range*. Farrar, Straus & Giroux, 1981.
Mellor, Anne K. *Mary Shelley: Her Life, Her Fiction, Her Monsters*. Methuen, 1988.
———. *Romanticism and Gender*. Routledge, 1993.
Miller, J. Hillis. *Topographies*. Stanford UP, 1995.
Milton, John. *Lycidas*. Harper & Row, 1966.
———. *Paradise Lost*. Norton, 2005.
Monsam, Angela. "Biography as Autopsy in William Godwin's Memoirs of the Author of 'A Vindication of the Rights of Woman.'" *Eighteenth-Century Fiction* 21.1 (2008), pp. 109–130.
Montesquieu, Charles de Secondat. *The Spirit of Laws*. Vol. 1, Dublin: Ewing & Faulkner, 1751.
Moody, Harry. *Aging: Concepts and Controversies*. 5th ed., Pine Forge, 2006.
Moretti, Franco. *The Way of the World: The Bildungsroman in European Culture*. Verso, 2000.
Mulvey-Roberts, Marie. *Gothic Immortals: The Fiction of the Brotherhood of the Rosy Cross*. Routledge, 1990.
———. "'A Physic Against Death': Eternal Life and the Enlightenment—Gender and Gerontology." *Literature and Medicine During the Eighteenth Century*, edited by Marie Mulvey-Roberts and Roy Porter, Routledge, 1993, pp. 151–167.
Mulvey-Roberts, Marie, and Roy Porter, eds. *Literature and Medicine During the Eighteenth Century*. Routledge, 1993.
Munich, Adrienne. *Queen Victoria's Secrets*. Columbia UP, 1998.
Murphy, Patricia. *Time is of the Essence: Temporality, Gender, and the New Woman*. SUNY P, 2001.
Musgrave, Richard. *Memoirs of the Different Rebellions in Ireland, From the Arrival of the English: Also, A Particular Detail of That Which Broke Out the 23d of May, 1798; With the History of the Conspiracy Which Preceded It*. Vol. 1, Dublin: Marchbank, 1802.
National Institutes of Health. "World's older population grows dramatically." 28 Mar. 2016, www.nih.gov/news-events/news-releases/worlds-older-population-grows-dramatically.
Needham, Gwendolyn B. "New Light on Maids 'Leading Apes in Hell.'" *The Journal of American Folklore* 75.296 (1962), pp. 106–119.

Nelson, Claudia. *Precocious Children & Childish Adults: Age Inversion in Victorian Literature.* Johns Hopkins UP, 2012.

Ni Chonaill, Siobhan. "'Why May Not Man One Day Be Immortal?': Population, Perfectibility, and the Ummortality Question in Godwin's Political Justice." *History of European Ideas* 33 (2007), pp. 25–39.

Niles, Lisa. "Malthusian Menopause: Aging and Sexuality in Elizabeth Gaskell's Cranford." *Victorian Literature and Culture* 33 (2005), pp. 293–310.

———. "Unproductive Productivity: Aging and Literature in the Nineteenth Century." Diss. Vanderbilt University, 2005.

Nordau, Max. *The Conventional Lies of Our Civilization.* Arno, 1975.

———. *Degeneration.* U of Nebraska P, 1993.

———. *Entartung.* Berlin: Carl Dunder, 1893.

Nunokawa, Jeff. "The Miser's Two Bodies: Silas Marner and the Sexual Possibilities of the Commodity." *Victorian Studies* 36.3 (1993), pp. 273–292.

Office for National Statistics (United Kingdom). "What does the 2011 Census tell us about older people." 6 Sep. 2013, www.ons.gov.uk/peoplepopulationandcommunity/birthsdeathsandmarriages/ageing/articles/whatdoesthe2011censustellusaboutolderpeople/2013-09-06.

Oppen, George. "Of Being Numerous." *New Collected Poems,* edited by Michael Davidson, New Directions, 2008, pp. 163–188.

Orwell, George. *The Collected Essays, Journalism, and Letters of George Orwell.* Edited by Sonia Orwell and Ian Angus. Harcourt, Brace and World, 1968.

Ottaway, Susannah R. *The Decline of Life: Old Age in Eighteenth-Century England.* Cambridge UP, 2004.

Owen, Wilfred. "Anthem for Doomed Youth." *First World War Poetry Digital Archive,* 4 May 2019, www.oucs.ox.ac.uk/ww1lit/collections/item/4891.

Paget, James. *Lectures on Nutrition, Hypertrophy, and Atrophy: Delivered in the Theatre of the Royal College of Surgeons,* May 1847. London: Wilson & Ogilvy, 1847.

Paley, Morton D. *Apocalypse and Millennium in English Romantic Poetry.* Oxford UP, 1999.

———. *Portraits of Coleridge.* Oxford UP, 1999.

Paul, C. Kegan. *William Godwin: His Friends and Contemporaries.* 2 vols, London: Henry S. King, 1876.

Paxton, Nancy. *George Eliot and Herbert Spencer: Feminism, Evolutionism and the Reconstruction of Gender.* Princeton UP, 1991.

Peacock, Thomas Love. *Melincourt: Or, Sir Oran Haut-ton.* Macmillan and Company, 1927.

Philp, Mark. *Godwin's Political Justice.* Duckworth, 1986.

Pick, Daniel. *Faces of Degeneration: A European Disorder, c. 1848–c. 1918.* Cambridge UP, 1989.

Plato. *Dialogues.* Vol. 1, edited by Benjamin Jowett, Clarendon, 1953.

Polwhele, Richard. *The Unsex'd Females: A Poem, Addressed to the Author of the Pursuits of Literature*. London: Printed for Cadell and Davies in the Strand, 1798.
Poovey, Mary. *The Proper Lady and the Woman Writer: Ideology as Style in the Works of Mary Wollstonecraft, Mary Shelley, and Jane Austen*. U of Chicago P, 1986.
Popper, Karl. *Conjectures and Refutations: The Growth of Scientific Knowledge*. Basic, 1965.
Port, Cynthia. "No Future? Aging, Temporality, History, and Reverse Chronologies." *Occasion: Interdisciplinary Studies in the Humanities* 4.31 (2012), pp. 1–19.
Porter, Roy. *Body Politic: Disease, Death, and Doctors in Britain, 1650–1900*. Cornell UP, 2001.
———. "Medical Futures." *Interdisciplinary Science Reviews* 26.1 (2001), pp. 35–42.
Praz, Mario. *The Romantic Agony*. 2nd ed., translated by Angus Davidson, Oxford UP, 1951.
Priestley, F.E.L. "Critical Introduction and Notes." *Enquiry Concerning Political Justice and its Influence on Modern Morals and Happiness*, vol. 3, edited by F.E.L. Priestley, U of Toronto P, 1946.
Pyle, Forest. "'Frail Spells': Shelley and the Ironies of Exile." *Romantic Circles*, Aug. 1999, n.p., www.rc.umd.edu/praxis/irony/pyle/frail.html.
Raitt, Suzanne. "Waste and Repair in Wilde's Dorian Gray." Interdisciplinary Nineteenth-Century Studies Conference (INCS), Pitzer College, Claremont, CA, 1 Apr. 2011.
Rajan, Tilottama. *Romantic Narrative: Shelley, Hays, Godwin, Wollstonecraft*. Johns Hopkins UP, 2010.
Rajan, Tilottama, and Julia Wright, eds. *Romanticism, History and the Possibilities of Genre: Re-forming Literature 1789–1837*. Cambridge UP, 1998.
Randel, Fred V. "The Political Geography of Horror in Mary Shelley's Frankenstein." *English Literary History* 70.2 (2003), pp. 465–491.
Richardson, Alan. "Erasmus Darwin and the Fungus School." *Wordsworth Circle* 33.3 (2002), pp. 113–116.
———. "Romanticism and the Body." *Literature Compass* 1.1 (2004), pp. 1–14.
Ricoeur, Paul. *Time and Narrative*. Translated by Kathleen Blamey and David Pellauer, U of Chicago P, 1990. 3 vols.
Robbins, Bruce. "The Cosmopolitan Eliot." *A Companion to George Eliot*, edited by Amanda Anderson and Harry E. Shaw, Wiley & Sons, 2013, pp. 400–412.
Rounce, Adam. "William Godwin: The Novel, Philosophy, and History." *History of European Ideas* 33 (2007), pp. 1–8.
Rousseau, Jean-Jacques. *The Confessions of J.J. Rousseau*. Belford, 1856.
Ruskin, John. *Sesame and Lilies: Lectures*. Arc Manor, 2008.
Rylance, Rick. *Victorian Psychology and British Culture, 1850–1880*. Oxford UP, 2000.

Schubert, Gotthilf Heinrich von. *Ansichten von der Nachtseite der Naturwissenschaft*. Wissenschaftliche Buchgesellschaft, 1967.

Sedgwick, Eve Kosofsky. *The Coherence of Gothic Conventions*. Arno, 1986.

Segal, Lynne. *Out of Time: The Pleasures and the Perils of Ageing*. Introduction by Elaine Showalter, Verso, 2013.

"senescence, n." *OED Online*, Oxford UP, 4 May 2019, www.oed.com/view/Entry/175887.

"The Seven Ages of Woman." *Pick-Me-Up* 18.444 (17 April 1897), p. 38.

"The Seven Ages of Woman (As Sir James Crichton Browne Seems Prophetically to See Them)." *Punch* 102 (14 May 1892), p. 231.

Shakespeare, William. *As You Like It*. *The Norton Shakespeare*, edited by Stephen Greenblatt, Walter Cohen, Jean E. Howard, and Katharine Eisaman Maus, 2nd ed., Norton, 2008.

———. *King Lear*. *The Norton Shakespeare*, edited by Stephen Greenblatt, Walter Cohen, Jean E. Howard, and Katharine Eisaman Maus, 2nd ed., Norton, 2008.

———. *The Tragedy of King Richard the Second*. *The Norton Shakespeare*, edited by Stephen Greenblatt, Walter Cohen, Jean E. Howard, and Katharine Eisaman Maus, 2nd ed., Norton, 2008.

———. *Richard III*. *The Norton Shakespeare*, edited by Stephen Greenblatt, Walter Cohen, Jean E. Howard, and Katharine Eisaman Maus, 2nd ed., Norton, 2008.

———. "Sonnets." *The Norton Shakespeare*, edited by Stephen Greenblatt, Walter Cohen, Jean E. Howard, and Katharine Eisaman Maus, 2nd ed., Norton, 2008.

Shaw, George Bernard. *Mrs. Warren's Profession*. Edited by Leonard Conolly, Broadview, 2005.

Shelley, Mary. *Frankenstein; Or, The Modern Prometheus*, Signet, 2000.

———. *The Last Man*. Edited by Anne Ruth McWhir, Broadview, 1996.

———. *The Life and Letters of Mary Wollstonecraft Shelley*. Edited by Mrs. Julian Marshall, vol. 2, Bentley & Son, 1889.

———. *Mathilda*. Edited by Janet Todd, Penguin, 2004.

———. *Valperga: Or, The Life and Adventures of Castruccio, Prince of Lucca*. Edited by Tilottama Rajan, Broadview, 1998.

Shelley, Percy Bysshe. "A Defence of Poetry." *Romantic Poetry and Prose*, edited by Harold Bloom and Lionel Trilling, Oxford UP, 1973, pp. 744–762.

———. *The Cenci: A Tragedy in Five Acts: An Authoritative Text Based on the 1819 Edition*. Edited by Cajsa C. Baldini, Valancourt, 2008.

———. *Prometheus Unbound, a Lyrical Drama in Four Acts with other Poems*. London: C. and J. Collier, 1820.

———. *Poetical Works*. Edited by Thomas Hutchinson, Oxford UP, 1970.

Shuttleworth, Sally. *George Eliot and Nineteenth Century Science: The Make-Believe of a Beginning*. Cambridge UP, 1986.

———. *The Mind of the Child: Child Development in Literature, Science, and Medicine, 1840–1900*. Oxford UP, 2010.

Silverman, Sam. "Trollope's The Fixed Period: A Nineteenth-Century Novel Revisited." *Illness, Crisis, and Loss* 12.4 (2004), pp. 272–283.

"The Silver Tsunami." *Economist*, 4 Feb. 2010, www.economist.com/business/2010/02/04/the-silver-tsunami.

Simpson, Jeffrey. "Our hospitals are not ready for the grey tsunami." *Globe and Mail*, 7 May 2018, www.theglobeandmail.com/opinion/our-hospitals-are-not-ready-for-the-grey-tsunami/article19113784/.

Small, Helen. *The Long Life*. Oxford UP, 2007.

Small, Helen, and Trudi Tate. *Literature, Science, Psychoanalysis 1830–1970: Essays in Honour of Gillian Beer*. Oxford UP, 2003.

Smalley, Donald Arthur, ed. *Anthony Trollope: The Critical Heritage*. Routledge, 1969.

Smith, Adam. *An Inquiry into the Nature and Causes of the Wealth of Nations*. Vol. 1, Dublin: Kelly, 1801.

Sonnenschein, Edward Adolf (E.A.). "Culture and Science." *Macmillan's Magazine* 53 (1886), pp. 5–16.

Spencer, Herbert. *Essays: Scientific, Political, Speculative*. Appleton, 1904.

———. *Herbert Spencer: An Autobiography*. Kessinger, 1904.

———. *The Principles of Biology*. Vol. 1, London: Williams and Norgate, 1864.

Statistics Canada. "Canada [Country] and Canada [Country] (table). Census Profile. 2016 Census." Statistics Canada Catalogue no. 98-316-X2016001. 29 Nov. 2017, www12.statcan.gc.ca/census-recensement/2016/dp-pd/prof/index.cfm?Lang=E.

Steinlight, Emily. *Populating the Novel: Literary Form and the Politics of Surplus Life*. Cornell UP, 2018.

Sterrenberg, Lee. "The Last Man: Anatomy of Failed Revolutions." *Nineteenth-Century Fiction* 33.3 (1978), pp. 324–347.

Stewart, Anthony Terence Quincey. *The Shape of Irish History*. McGill-Queens UP, 2001.

Stockwell, Peter. "Introduction." *Impossibility Fiction: Alternativity, Extrapolation, Speculation*, edited by Derek Littlewood and Peter Stockwell, Rodopi, 1996.

Strickland, Agnes. *The Seven Ages of Woman: and Other Poems*. London: Hurst and Chance, 1827.

Swift, Jonathan. *Gulliver's Travels*. *The Norton Anthology of British Literature*, 5th ed., pp. 915–1077.

Swinburne, Algernon Charles. "La Soeur de la Reine." *New Writings by Swinburne*, edited by Cecil Y. Lang, Syracuse UP, 1964, pp. 103–118.

Swinnen, Aagje, and Cynthia Port. "Aging, Narrative, and Performance: Essays from the Humanities." *International Journal of Ageing and Later Life* 7 (2012), pp. 9–15.

Thane, Pat. *Old Age in English History*. Oxford UP, 2000.

———. "Social Histories of Old Age and Ageing." *Journal of Social History* 37.1 (2003), pp. 93–111.

Thompson, Derek. "What Are Young Non-Working Men Doing?" *Atlantic*, 25 July 2016, www.theatlantic.com/business/archive/2016/07/what-are-young-non-working-men-doing/492890/.

Thompson, G.R. "Introduction: Romanticism and the Gothic Tradition." *Gothic Imagination: Essays in Dark Romanticism*, edited by G.R. Thompson., Washington State UP, 1974.

Trollope, Anthony. *The Fixed Period*. Norilana, 2008.

United Nations. "Ageing." 15 Dec. 2018, www.un.org/en/sections/issues-depth/ageing/.

United States Census Bureau. "Age & Sex Tables" (2016). 15 Dec. 2018. www.census.gov/topics/population/age-and-sex/data/tables.html.

"V21 Forum on Strategic Presentism." *Victorian Studies* 59.1 (2016), pp. 87–126.

Vesalius, Andreas. *On the Fabric of the Human Body. Book I: The Bones and Cartilages*. Trans. William Frank Richardson and John Burd Carman. San Francisco: Norman, 1998.

Vickers, Neil. *Coleridge and the Doctors 1795–1806*. Oxford UP, 2004.

———. "Thomas Beddoes and the German Psychological Tradition." *Notes and Records of the Royal Society* 63.3 (2009), pp. 311–321.

Von Schlun, Betsy. "William Godwin's St. Leon and the Fatal Legacy of Alchemy." *The Golden Egg: Alchemy in Art and Literature*, edited by Alexandra Lembert and Elmar Schenkel. Galda and Wilch, 2002.

Vrettos, Athena. *Somatic Fictions: Imagining Illness in Victorian Culture*. Stanford UP, 1995.

Wagner, Tamara Silvia. "The Miser's New Notes and the Victorian Sensation Novel: Plotting the Magic of Paper Money." *Victorian Review* 31.2 (2005), pp. 79–98.

Wallace, Jennifer. "Keats's Frailty: The Body and Biography." *Romantic Biography*, edited by Arthur Bradley and Alan Rawes, Ashgate, 2002, pp. 139–151.

Wallace, Robert. *A Dissertation on the Numbers of Mankind: In Ancient and Modern Times*. A. Constable and Company, 1809.

Watt, Ian P. *The Rise of the Novel: Studies in Defoe, Richardson, and Fielding*. U of California P, 2001.

Wells, H.G. *War of the Worlds*. Edited by David Yerkes Hughes and Harry M. Geduld, Indiana UP, 1993.

Wilde, Oscar. *The Complete Works Of Oscar Wilde: The Picture of Dorian Gray: The 1890 and 1891 Texts*, vol. 3, Oxford UP, 2005.

———. "Literary and Other Notes." *Woman's World*, vol. 1, Cassel and Company, 1888, pp. 132–136.

Williams, Cynthia Schoolar. "Mary Shelley's Bestiary: The Last Man and the Discourse of Species." *Literature Compass* 3.2 (2006), pp. 138–148.

Williams, Sherwood. "The Rise of a New Degeneration: Decadence and Atavism in Vandover and the Brute." *English Literary History* 57.3 (1990), pp. 709–736.

Williamson, George. "Mutability, Decay, and Seventeenth-Century Melancholy." *English Literary History* 2.2 (1935), pp. 121–150.

Winyard, Ben, and Holly Furneaux. "Dickens, Science, and the Victorian Literary Imagination." *19: Interdisciplinary Studies in the Long Nineteenth Century* 10 (2010), pp. 1–17.
Wollstonecraft, Mary. *A Vindication of the Rights of Woman*. Edited by Marian Brody, Penguin, 2004.
Woodward, Kathleen. *Aging and its Discontents: Freud and Other Fictions*. Indiana UP, 1991.
———. "Assisted Living: Aging, Old Age, Memory, Aesthetics." *Occasion: Interdisciplinary Studies in the Humanities* 4.31 (2012), pp. 1–13.
———. *At Last, the Real Distinguished Thing: The Late Poems of Eliot, Pound, Stevens and Williams*. Ohio State UP, 1980.
———. *Statistical Panic: Cultural Politics and Poetics of the Emotions*. Duke UP, 2009.
———, ed. *Figuring Age: Women, Bodies, Generations*. Indiana UP, 1999.
Wordsworth, William. *The Poetical Works of Wordsworth*. Edited by Thomas Hutchinson, Oxford UP, 1960.
———. *The Prelude: A Parallel Text*. Edited by J.C. Maxwell, Penguin, 1971.
World Bank. "Population ages 65 and above (% of total) (2017). 15 Dec. 2018, data.worldbank.org/indicator/SP.POP.65UP.TO.ZS.
World Health Organization. "Ageing and Health." 5 Feb. 2018, www.who.int/newsroom/fact-sheets/detail/ageing-and-health.
Wrigley E.A., and R.S. Schofield. *The Population History of England, 1541–1871: A Reconstruction*. Harvard UP, 1982.
Youngquist, Paul. *Monstrosities: Bodies and British Romanticism*. U of Minnesota P, 2003.
Zwierlein, Anne. "'Exhausting the Powers of Life': Aging, Energy, and Productivity in Nineteenth-Century Scientific and Literary Discourses." *Interdisciplinary Perspectives on Ageing in Nineteenth-Century Culture*, edited by Katharina Boehm, Anna Farkas, and Anne Zwierlein, Routledge, 2013, pp. 38–56.

Index

Aesop, 80, 95
age, aging, and older age: abuse of (elder abuse), 159n3; accelerated, advanced, or premature, xxxi, 41, 52, 55, 66, 74, 117, 119; aesthetics of, xxiv, xl–xli, 11, 61, 64, 111, 133, 138–139; affects of poverty on, 117–119, 122, 127, 129, 152n8; "age anxiety" (anxiety about), 165n15; ageism (prejudice against) and stigmatizing of, xli, 7–9, 81, 99, 139, 146–148; "age stamp" (indicators or identity) of, 33, 105, 113–114, 117, 125–127, 135, 138; alchemy used in, 1–2, 18, 23–26, 46, 129, 137, 156n18, 157n22; *elixir vitae*, 15, 21–22, 27–29, 31; anti-aging culture and "industry," 19, 81, 148, 165n15; biological necessity of, xx, 3, 13, 20, 23–26, 30, 56; biopoliticization of, xix–xxv, xxxvi, xliv, 3, 13, 16, 19, 30, 60, 115, 148, 154n10; community sense of, 52; counterfeiting in, 101–103, 110–114, 126–127, 132–137, 146, 159n8, 163n6, 165n15; crisis associated with, xix, 62, 147; demographic containment of, 143–147; diseases and disabilities (physical and mental) of, 112, 141–142, 162n21; aridity or impotence, 95, 161n18; dementia (including Alzheimer's), 104, 112, 139, 142, 162n21, 163n3; senility ("senile diseases"), xliv, 101–107, 111–112, 139, 163n7; economic stability of, 118, 121, 127; elimination of: by "escape," 31; by immortality, 3–4, 11, 13–14, 20–23, 26–28, 153nn2–3, 154n8; by prolongation or prolongevity, 8–10, 13–16, 66, 151n3, 153n2, 153n5, 154n8, 155nn15–16; ephebiphobia in (fear or dislike of youth), xxxii, xxxv, 34–40, 48–51, 81, 90, 143, 158n6; equivalency of the terms "age" and "aging," xxxii; euthanasia in, 74, 143; financial cost of, 94, 118–119, 129, 144; geriatrics, xii, 114; geronticide (elder murder), xliii, 42, 46, 144–146, 159n3, 164n11; gerontology, 64; gerontophilia, xxxiv–xxxv, 39; Godwin-Malthus debate on, xix–xxi, xxvii, 2, 54, 147; health policy on, 161n17; intellectual intervention into: in narrative fictionality or literary representations, xix–xxi, xxiii, xxxviii, xl, xlii, 20, 30–31, 34, 94, 132–133, 146–149, 161n17; in

age, aging, and older age *(continued)* speculation, 16–20, 30, 156n18; interconnection of disciplinary knowledges about, xxxviii, 17, 20, 141–143; intergenerationality of (coexistence, dialectic, miscegenation, simultaneity, and/or synthesis with youth), xliv, 45, 53–58, 62, 67, 73–78, 83–85, 90–96, 99, 102, 122, 127, 134, 149, 161n18; life expectancy (or lifespan or lifecourse) of, xxiii, xxix, xxxii, xlii, 13, 30–33, 72, 121–122, 142, 149, 151n3, 160n13; class differences in, xxii–xxiii, 152n6, 152n8; loneliness and isolation of, 55, 119, 162n21; meaning to young people of, xi–xii; medical, medicalized, and/or scientific thought about, xxi–xxii, xxv–xxvi, xxviii, xxxix, xli–xlii, xliv, 3, 5, 14–21, 30–31, 64–66, 72–73, 103, 114, 139, 147, 154n10, 156n17, 161n17, 163n7; the mind (thinking principle) as a factor in, 8, 11–12, 19; moralized physical traits of, 10–11; optimism and idealism about, 141; physiological virtues of, 51; productive imaginary of, 55; readers' awareness of, xi–xiii, xliii–xliv, 22–23, 32, 79, 96, 135, 148; reanimation in, 73–77; relationship to war of, 147; "second childhood" of, xxxv, 110; in soldiers, 131–132; suicide in, 146

age, aging, and older age: conceptualizations of: as an analytical category of textual study, xxii, 36, 148; as a conditional state, xx, xxv, 30–31, 74, 142; as diseased or disgusting excess or economical waste, 65, 159n3; in the Enlightenment, xx, 6–8, 13, 16; in evolutionary approaches, 73; in geological metaphors, 70–72, 95, 104, 162n22; as gravitational phenomenology, 8, 10; as the graying of society, xli; as helpless, 92; as heterogeneous, 70, 72; in iconography, images and thematics, xl, 64; as inexorable, 92; as influenced by aesthetics of embodiment, 65; *Lebenstreppe* model ("steps of life"), xxxvi–xxxvii, 70, 108; as a linear progression of stages, xxiv, xxxvi–xxxix, 12, 14, 70, 142, 151n3, 154n10, 160n13; as a means of survival, 51; as a miserly condition, 79–80, 83, 94, 159n8, 162n19; in organicist metaphors, 72–75, 119, 160n9, 161nn15–16; as paradoxical or double-stranded, xxxi, 53, 58, 143, 149; as perverse and malignant, 41; as physiological waste (entropy), xliv, 65–69, 74–87, 94–97, 118, 122, 143, 159n3, 161n16; population-based, xxvi, xxxvi, xl, 31, 46–48, 59, 104–106, 114–116, 122–123, 144–147, 151n3; reflecting affective states and social conditions, xxxvii; religious, xxi, xxv; secular, xxiii; as senescence, xli, 51–53, 61, 106, 129, 151n3; as social dis-ease and evolutionary decline, 8, 102, 160n10, 165n15; as a social ideal, 37; as socially renovating, 53, 143; in terms of lastness, 52, 55, 61; in terms of lateness, 61; terrestrial visions of, 69; as threatened by youth (intergenerational conflict), xxv, xxxiv, 34, 38–39, 134, 149, 152n10; "trauma of solidification" in, 71; using topographical language, 104–105, 138, 143, 160n11;

as a voluntary process, 12–13; mentioned, xxi–xxix, xxxiv–xxxix, xli–xliv, 4, 31, 67–74, 104, 138–146, 151n3, 160n13

Age (or "Aging") Studies, xii, 61; definition of, xxi; gender issues in, 104–107, 125–128, 152n8, 163n3; history of, xxii, 155n13; influence of Benjamin on, xiii; interdisciplinarity of, xxii, 148; narrative approaches to, xlii, 30, 147; perspective on "crisis" of humanities, xlii; queer temporalities and subjectivities in, 103, 128, 137, 163n4; scope of, xxi, 148; terms and ideas in, xxxii, 139; use of demographic data in, xxii–xxiii, xxvi; value for reading Victorian novels of, 66

alchemy. *See* age, aging, and older age

Alighieri, Dante, 23, 25, 156n20

Alzheimer, Louis, 139

American Revolution, 152n10

Aristophanes, 87, 90, 127

Aristotle, 14, 142, 157n2, 161n18

Arnold, Matthew, xi, xiii, xix, xxi, 141–143, 149

Austen, Jane, 136

Barbauld, Anna Letitia, 113

Baudelaire, Charles, 102

Beddoes, Thomas, 15, 156n17

Beer, Gillian, 73

Benjamin, Walter, xiii, 110

Bewell, Alan, 7, 36

Blackwood, John, 76, 90

Blake, William, xxxiv, 9, 10, 33, 57, 85–87

Bloom, Harold, 98, 132

Bosch, Hieronymus, 81

Breughel, Pieter, the Elder, 81–82

British Medical Journal, 112

Brogden, Mike, 42, 159n3

Browning, Robert, 63, 98, 141–142

Buckley, Chris, 146

Burke, Edmund, xxv, xxxiv–xxxv, xliii, 15, 22, 39, 40, 46, 48, 57, 59, 102, 148, 153nn13–14, 154n9

Burney, Fanny, 113

Butler, Samuel, 146, 154n7

Byron, George Gordon, Lord, 33, 38, 52–53, 157n4, 159n1

Carlyle, Thomas, 62, 68

Carroll, Lewis, 94, 98, 108

Catholic Emancipation movement, 42

Charcot, Jean-Martin, 112, 114, 163n7

Chase, Karen, xii, xxiii, 55, 64, 66, 74, 108, 135, 161n17

the Child: as a capitalized figure, 103

Cicero, xxxv, 14, 80, 153n14, 161n18

Cohen, William A., xxxvii, 65, 159n3

Cole, Thomas R., xii, xxxvi, 155nn12–13, 155n15, 160n13

Coleridge, Samuel Taylor, xxxvi, 155n15–16

Coleridge, Sara, 62

Collins, Wilkie, 98

counterfeiting. *See* age, aging, and older age

Crichton-Browne, James, 112, 134

Crimean war, 131

Cruikshank, Margaret, xxxii, 104, 144, 146

D., Auguste, 139

Dames, Nicholas, xxxviii

Darwin, Charles, 26, 62, 64, 71–72, 74, 95, 119, 135, 148, 159n3, 162n2

Darwin, Erasmus, 26–29, 31, 154n11

de Beauvoir, Simone, xxii, 154n10, 155n15

dementia (including Alzheimer's). *See* age, aging, and older age: diseases and disabilities of

De Quincey, Thomas, 44–46, 50, 57, 62, 159n1
Descartes, René, 6, 7, 19
Dickens, Charles, xii, 65, 74, 80–81, 98, 108, 121, 108, 159n3, 161n17
disability studies, 61
Donne, John, 113, 135

Edelman, Lee, 103
Ehrenreich, Barbara, xxi
Eliot, George: influence of: Blake, 86, 93; Browne, 98; Burke, 74; Dutch masters, 81; Lewes, 66–68, 75–79, 83, 85, 93, 159n5, 161n16; Malthus, 75; P. Shelley, 93; Plato, 87, 90; W. Wordsworth, 90–92; *Adam Bede*, 81; *Daniel Deronda*, 75–77, 92, 96–97, 108; *Life and Letters*, 78; *Middlemarch*, 75–76, 80, 86–87, 92–99, 136; restoration of Romanticism in, 98; *Scenes of Clerical Life*, 75; *Silas Marner*, xliii–xliv, 66–67, 73–87, 90–99, 102–104, 122, 162nn19–21, 162n22; mentioned, 62, 161n17
the Enlightenment: conceptions of the body as a mechanical instrument (*homme-machine*), 6–8, 16, 22; ideals of perpetuity, xx, 12–15, 20; influences of, 154n6, 154n8; perceptions of human lifespan, xx
Enquiry Concerning Political Justice (Godwin), xix–xx, 2–8, 11–15, 20, 26–27, 31–33, 37, 53, 153n1, 153n4, 154n9, 154n11; "Of Health, and the Prolongation of Human Life," 8–10, 13–23, 28–30, 114, 153n2, 153n5, 154n8, 154n10, 209
ephebiphobia. *See* age, aging, and older age
euthanasia. *See* age, aging, and older age

feminism, 36, 124, 136; critiques of, 112–113; protofeminist emancipation, 115, 117
fin de siècle. *See* the Victorian Age and the Victorians
First World War, 147
Fitzgerald, F. Scott, 146
Flourens, Jean-Pierre, xlii, 72
Foucault, Michel, xxi, 159n2
Franklin, Benjamin, xxx, 6
Freud, Sigmund, 68, 133, 163n7

Galen, 14
Gallagher, Catherine, xxix, xxxi, xxxiii, 19–20, 65, 75
Gaskell, Elizabeth, xxxiii, 75, 153n12
geriatrics. *See* age, aging, and older age
gerontophilia. *See* age, aging, and older age
geronticide. *See* age, aging, and older age
gerontology. *See* age, aging, and older age
Gillray, James, 42
Gissing, George: influences on: Ruskin, 130; Tennyson, 130–131; *The Nether World*, 110–111, 116; *New Grub Street*, 116, 118, 120, 164n9; *The Odd Women*, xliv, 105, 114–133, 138, 145, 164n9, 164nn11–12; "The Place of Realism in Fiction," 124
Godwin, William: basic error of claims of, 14; compared to Hume, 12, 154n7; concept of the mind as the body's perpetual engine, 8; fall from public favor of, 14; father figure of Romantic "medical imagination," 5; incipient Romanticism of, 12; influence on twenty-first-century writings of, xliv; links between literary and philosophical writing,

2–3; member of Johnson's dissenting circle, 5, 15, 154n11, 156n17; personal library of, 156n17; psychological realism of, 154n6; repugnancy for involuntary fixity of, 12; shift in thinking about the meaning of aging of, 3; utopian optimism about the prolongation of life of, 13, 16, 18; diary of, 156n17; *The Enquirer*, 5; *Enquiry Concerning Political Justice*, xix–xx, xxix, 2–15, 20, 26–37, 53, 107, 153n1, 153n4, 154n9, 154n11; "Of Health, and the Prolongation of Human Life," 2–23, 28–30, 114, 153n2, 153n5, 154n8, 154n10; *Essay on Sepulchres*, 52; *Memoirs of Mary Wollstonecraft*, 5; *Of Population*, 53–54; *St. Leon*, xx, 1–5, 13–33, 40, 60, 65, 126, 135, 153nn2–3, 154n11, 156n18, 156n22; *Things as They Are; or The Adventures of Caleb Williams*, xx, 2, 5; *Thoughts Occasioned by the Perusal of Dr. Parr's Spital Sermon*, 20, 53, 156n19; mentioned, xxv, xxx, xliii, 34, 39, 41, 46, 53, 58, 143
Godwin-Malthus debate, xix–xxi, xxvii, 2, 54, 147, 158n5
Goethe, Johann Wolfgang von, xxiv, 15, 42
Grand, Sarah, 163n8
Gruman, Gerald J., 15, 151n3, 155n13, 155n15
Gullette, Margaret, xi, xxi, xii, xxxii, 30, 160n10

Haggard, H. Rider, 135
Hall, G. Stanley, xli
Hardy, Thomas, xii, 74, 119, 129, 138, 160n10
Hayflick, Leonard, xli
Hazlitt, William, xxxvi, 154n9

Heath, Kay, xii, 66, 161n18, 165n15
Heath, William, 42
Heringman, Noah, 71
Hippocrates, 14
Hufeland, Christoph Wilhelm, 15–19, 23, 31, 66, 72, 154n8, 155nn15–16, 156n17
humanities: "crisis" of, xlii; relevance of, xliii; "strategic presentism" in, xliii, 153n16
Hume, David, xxvii, 12, 154n7
Hunt, Leigh, xxxiii
Huxley, Aldous, 146
hysteria. *See* women

ideopathology, 7
infanticide, xxviii, 153n12
Ishiguro, Kazuo, 146

Jameson, Fredric, 25, 151n3
Jenner, Edward, 155n15

Kant, Immanuel, 15, 160n9, 161n16
Katz, Stephen, xii, 104, 155n15, 163n3, 163n7
Keats, John, 61, 63–65, 138, 155n15
King, Amy M., xxx, 161n18
Kipling, Rudyard, 131–133, 164n12
Kornbluh, Anna, 147
Kristeva, Julia, 106–107, 163n5, 164n10

Lamb, Charles, 61
Landor, Walter Savage, 61
Lebenskraft ("vital power" or "life force"), 15–16
Lebenstreppe. *See* age, aging, and older age: conceptualizations of
Lewes, George Henry, xliii–xliv, 66–78, 83–85, 95, 159n5, 159n7, 161nn15–17
Linnaeus, Carl, xxx

Looser, Devoney, xii
Lukács, George, 151n2
Lyell, Charles, 70–71, 75, 95

Malthus, Thomas Robert: *An Essay on the Principle of Population*, xix–xx, xxiv–xxxvi, 2, 20, 33, 39–53, 59, 97, 106, 148, 151n1, 156n19, 157n4, 158n5; Malthusianism, 38, 47–48, 58–59, 75, 115, 119, 127–128; anti-Malthusian backlash, 34; "Malthusian crisis," 56; Malthusian ephebiphobia, 81, 151n1; Malthusian paradigm shift, 65; Malthusian realism in twenty-first-century writings, xliv; Malthusian themes in Gaskell, 153n12; optimism about older age, 35; portrayal of the poor, 40, 151n1; review of Godwin's *Of Population*, 54; skepticism of youth, xliii, 36, 151n1; mentioned, 42, 52, 57, 120, 157n3
Mangum, Teresa, xii, 66, 94
Mann, Thomas, 136
Marcet, Jane, xxxiii
Martineau, Harriet, xxxiii, 61
Maturin, Charles, 30
McLane, Maureen N., xxv, 26, 39, 47, 157n5
McManners, John, 52
McPhee, John, 160n12
Mellor, Anne K., 38, 157n2, 157n4
men: fecundity and masculinity of, xxxiii, 39, 49, 106–107, 113, 125
Mentor, Lillian Frances, 146
Merleau-Ponty, Maurice, 90
Middleton, Thomas, 146, 164n11
Miller, J. Hillis, 104, 160n11, 163n4
Milton, John, 39, 78, 80
misogyny. *See* women
Mizumara, Minae, 146

modernism, 146
Moretti, Franco, xxiv, 34
Morgan, Benjamin, 147

Napoleon Bonaparte, 42
Nelson, Claudia, 66, 108, 120–121
Newton, Isaac, 8
Niles, Lisa, 75, 128
Nordau, Max, 101–107, 111, 126, 137, 162nn1–2, 165n15
Norris, Frank, 103
the novel: as the best mode of literature to address human aging, xxxviii; elusive form of, 20; foundational claim of, 19–20; influence on readers of, 96, 124; as a key resource for exploring human nature and the body, xli; portrayal of youth in, 34; realism in, xliv, 124, 128; socially disruptive economies in, 22

Oppen, George, 148–149
organicism, 72–75, 119, 160n9, 161nn15–16
the Orient: associations with sexual reproduction, xxviii, 45, 47; temporal longevity of, 44
Orwell, George, 116–117, 164n9
Ottaway, Susannah, xxii, 155n13, 155n15
Ovid, 42
Owen, Wilfred, 146–147

Paine, Tom, 154n9
Paley, Morton D., 53, 153n13
Patmore, Coventry, 107
Peacock, Thomas Love, 40
Pick-Me-Up, 112–113
Pitt, William, the Younger, xxxvi
plague, 36–41, 48–58, 150, 157n1
Plato, 87, 111

Polwhele, Richard, 113
Ponce de León, Juan, 14
Poor Laws, xxvii, 148
Poovey, Mary, xxxii, 36, 158n5
Popper, Karl, 17–18
population: biological and genealogical principles of, xxxvi; body-nation analogy of, xxxi, 59; as a character in the cultural landscape, xxi, xxiv; concept of "overpopulation," xxix, 45–48; control of, xxviii–xxix; defining experience of nineteenth-century life, 151n2; growth of, xxx–xxxiii, 152nn4–5; literature about and studies of, xxvii–xxviii
Punch, 111–112

queer theory, 103, 105, 128, 137, 163n4

Radcliffe, Ann, 30, 113
Raitt, Suzanne, 66–67, 159n6
Ricoeur, Paul, 59
Roman Catholicism, 42, 48
Romanticism and the Romantics: aging of, 63–64, 98; association with the supernatural, 5, 158n7; concerns about nation and empire, 44; dark, 34, 61, 158n7; frail, xliii, 34, 60–62, 90–92, 143; geological metaphors in, 71; ideas of the imagination, 11; influence of medicine and science on, 5, 155n15, 155n17; intermingling of youth and age in, 44; materialism of, 12, 154n11; "mode" in writing, 18; suspicion of modern economic life, 69; suspicion of the past, 41; youth model in, 33–34, 42, 46, 57, 61–64, 90, 99, 148
Rousseau, Jean-Jacques, xx, 14, 23
Rowley, William, 164n11

Ruskin, John, 107–110, 117–118, 120, 123–127, 130, 132

Sedgwick, Eve Kosofsky, 29, 163n4
Segal, Lynne, 103
senescence. *See* age, aging, and older age: conceptualizations of
senility. *See* age, aging, and older age: diseases and disabilities of
sexuality: asexual reproduction, 26–29; associations with the Orient, xxviii, 45, 47; "botanical vernacular" for, xxx–xxxi, xxxi; homosexuality, 103
Shakespeare, William: *King Lear*, xi, xxv, 8, 53, 80, 97, 105, 118, 164n11; *The Merchant of Venice*, 80; *Much Ado About Nothing*, 113; Sonnet 63, 50; Sonnet 129, 65; *The Taming of the Shrew*, 113; *The Tragedy of King Richard the Second*, 93; *The Winter's Tale*, 37, 76; *As You Like It*, xxiv, xxxi, 109, 112–113
Shaw, George Bernard, xxv, xli, 133–134151n3
Shelley, Mary: influence of: Byron, 38; Godwin, 39–40, 52–53, 58, 60; Malthus, 39–40, 47–48, 51–53, 58–59, 158n5; Milton, 39; Percy Shelley, 40; Wollstonecraft, 37; Young, 52; personal life of: idealization of her husband, 58; loyalty to her father, 41–42; treatment of by her father-in-law, 42; feminist readings of, 36; *Frankenstein*, 35, 40, 46–50, 158nn5–6; *The Last Man*, xliii, 34–42, 46–63, 90, 96, 107, 115, 147, 158n5; *The Life and Letters of Mary Wollstonecraft Shelley*, 34; *Mathilda*, 35, 40–41; the role of aging and old age in, 35; *Valperga*, 35, 40–41

Shelley, Percy Bysshe: "Promethean politics" of, 38; "Alastor; or, The Spirit of Solitude," v, 46, 149; *The Cenci*, 11; "A Defence of Poetry," 11, 33, 38, 157n2; "England 1819," 41; "Ode to the West Wind," 11; "Peter Bell the Third," 63; *Prometheus Unbound*, 47, 157n3; "The Revolt of Islam," 157n3; mentioned, xxvi, xliii, 5, 34, 42, 52, 57–58, 98, 157n4, 159n1
Shuttleworth, Sally, xxxviii, 75, 159n5, 161n16
Small, Helen, xii, 30, 68, 155n13
Smith, Adam, xxvii, xxviii, xxx, 45, 154n7
Sophocles, xxv
Southey, Robert: xxxvi, 98
Spencer, Herbert, 68, 156n21, 161n16
Steinlight, Emily, xxv, 158n5
Stevenson, Robert Louis, xli, 80, 103
Strickland, Agnes, 109–112, 132
suicide. *See* age, aging, and older age
Swift, Jonathan, 11, 53
Swinburne, Algernon Charles, 108

Tait's Edinburgh Magazine, 62
Tenniel, John, 158n6
Tennyson, Alfred, Lord, 122, 126, 130, 131–132, 141, 164n12
Thane, Pat, xxii, 152n4, 152n10
Trollope, Anthony, xliv, 62, 65, 74, 143–146, 159n3, 159n4, 164n11

Vesalius, Andreas, 68
Victoria, Queen, 64, 98, 108, 135
the Victorian Age and the Victorians: adult female subjectivity in, 108, 110, 137; aged misers in literature of, 79–80, 83, 94–95, 162n19; ageism in, 99; aging of, 64, 67, 137–138; associations with older age in, 98, 161n17; counterfeit progress in, 114–116, 128–129, 133, 135; critiques of the Romantics in, 98–99; cult of domesticity ("separate spheres") in, 106, 110; cult of the invalid in, 61, 158n9; evolutionary thought in, 73–74; exploitation of natural resources in, 72, 75; *fin de siècle* literary writing in, 101–39; gender and temporality in, 107, 110, 119–120, 125–128, 152n8; genre of illness in, 61; iconography of Queen Victoria in, 108; idea of "economy of the body" in, 68–69; ideas of waste and repair in, 65–69, 74–87, 94–97, 118, 122, 143, 159n3, 161n16; imagination of aging in, 66; inception of "the elderly subject" in, 64; interest in linkages of youth and age in, xliii, 65, 99; the longevity narrative in, xx, 31, 105, 138–139, 142, 151n3; marriage in, 126–129; masquerade in, 136; misogyny in, 99; motherhood in, 121; organicisim in, 72–75, 119, 160n9, 161nn15–16; self-fashioning of, 64, 98; senile topography of, 104–105, 138, 143, 160n11; skepticism about, 133; thermodynamic hypothesis of life in, 68

waste and repair. *See* the Victorian Age and the Victorians: ideas of
Watt, Ian, 34
Wells, H.G., 7
Wilde, Oscar, 65, 74, 103, 126, 159n8, 164n13
Wollstonecraft, Mary, 5, 37, 113, 154n11
women: "age stamp" (indicators or identity) of, 33, 105, 113–114,

117, 125–127, 135, 138; aging of, 104–105, 108–110, 132, 135, 163n3; alignment with soldiers of, 131; Alzheimer's dementia (AD) in, 163n3; as angel-women, 107, 132, 165n14; anti-feminism, 112–113; "cerebral physiology" of, 112; childbirth of, 163n8; as counterfeiting, aping, or odd, 110–114, 121–130, 134–137, 163n6, 163n8; economic potential of, 124, 129; fecundity of, xxxii–xxxiv, 42, 120; female subjectivity, 108, 110, 112, 116, 135, 137; hysteria in, 163n7; ideal feminine in, 107–108; masculine style of, 125; mild cognitive impairment (MCI) in, 163n3; misogyny (dislike of and prejudice against), 99, 106, 112–113; as monster women, 165n14; motherhood of, xxxiii, 110, 121; as the New Woman, 105–107, 110, 112–115, 130, 165n14, 110l; parodies of, 111–113; portrayal of in fiction, 94; redundancy of, 106, 127, 130–131; reproductive futurism of, 103–104, 134–135, 163n8; role of literature in progress of, 130; ruling capacity of, 118, 165n14; second motherhood of, 110; senility ("senile diseases") in, 163n7; sexual relationships of, 163n8; spinsterhood of, xxxii–xxxiii, 106, 110, 114–116, 122, 163n8; temporality and, 107, 112–113, 125–128; the "Woman Question," xliv, 104–105, 115–117, 135; womenchildren (or child-women, or girl-women) in novels, 108, 120–123, 126, 129; work of, 124, 128–129; youth in, 109
Woodward, Kathleen, xl, xii, 104, 136, 165n15

Wordsworth, Dorothy, 61
Wordsworth, William: as a character in a play, 108; public reputation of, 159n1; "Animal Tranquility and Decay," 62; "Intimations of Immortality from Recollections of Early Childhood," 12–13; *Lyrical Ballads*, 63; "Michael," 90–92, 99; *The Prelude*, 33; "Resolution and Independence," xlii, 40, 62, 71–74, 79, 98; "Simon Lee," 62; "Sonnet Composed Upon Westminster Bridge," 73; "Sonnet to an Octogenarian," 62; "The Fountain," 79–80; "The Old Cumberland Beggar," 62; "The World is Too Much With Us," 69; mentioned, xii, xxvi, xli, 40, 61, 76, 154n9

Young, Edward, 52
youth: as an internal enemy of age, xxxiv; as antithetical to an *ancien régime*, xxvi, 42; association with hope and progress, 51, 129; "as the most meaningful part of life," xxiv; compared to plague, 50, 157n1; counterfeit of, 101–103, 110–114, 126–127, 132–137, 146, 159n8, 163n6, 165n15; disastrous potential of, 34, 48–51; "elasticity" of, 10; ephebiphobia (fear or dislike of), xxxii, xxxv, 34–40, 48–51, 81, 90, 143, 158n6; idealization of, xliii, 33–34, 42, 46, 57, 61–64, 90, 99, 148; intergenerationality of (coexistence, dialectic, miscegenation, simultaneity, and synthesis with old age), xliv, 45, 53–58, 62, 67, 73–78, 83–85, 90–96, 99, 102, 122, 127, 134, 149, 161n18; meaning of older age to, xi–xii; as a miserly condition, 81, 159n8; optimism of, 102,

youth *(continued)*
122; pessimism of, 129; primacy of, 136; as a relic of the past, 45; reproductive capacity of, xxix, xxxi, 34; skepticism about, 36, 42, 151n1; in soldiers, 132; tastes and attitudes of, 23; waste and repair in, 65–69, 74–75, 97, 143

Zola, Émile, 65, 101

www.ingramcontent.com/pod-product-compliance
Lightning Source LLC
Chambersburg PA
CBHW030647230426
43665CB00011B/990